FrameWork

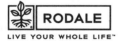

Every day our brands connect with and inspire millions of
people to live a life of the mind, body, spirit — a whole life.

FrameWork

YOUR 7-STEP PROGRAM FOR
HEALTHY MUSCLES, BONES, AND JOINTS

NICHOLAS A. DiNUBILE, MD

with WILLIAM PATRICK

RODALE

MORE PRAISE FOR *FrameWork:*

"During my 21-year major league career it was amazing to see the advances in training and medicine from the time I first made it to the big leagues in 1981 to the time I retired in 2001. Dr. DiNubile's book is a striking example of that and how a firm understanding of your body and how best to keep it in shape can enhance every part of your life. Having gone through my share of injuries from bumps and bruises to a herniated disk, I wish that resources like *FrameWork* were available to me throughout my career."

—CAL RIPKEN, JR.
Baseball's all-time "Iron Man," two-time AL MVP, nineteen-time All-Star (including two-time All-Star Game MVP), two-time Golden Glove recipient, longest consecutive-games-played streak in baseball history (2,632 games)

"Dr. DiNubile, a renowned orthopaedic surgeon, is a sports medicine specialist whose expertise in physical fitness parallels his leadership in the medical profession. As physician for both the Philadelphia 76ers and the Pennsylvania Ballet, Dr. DiNubile is the master of preventive medicine for the musculoskeletal system. His new book, *FrameWork,* clearly presents his comprehensive seven-step program for healthy muscles, bones, and joints that enhance your frame durability and enable you to live stronger longer. Dr. DiNubile's highly effective approach for avoiding injuries and delaying degenerative problems is the missing knowledge/application link that those of us in the fitness field have been long awaiting. Without question, this well-researched and superbly written book represents the future of personal fitness, with a practical exercise plan that will definitely exceed your expectations, especially if you previously have tried other physical fitness or sports conditioning programs. I can think of no other book that I recommend more highly for exercisers and sports enthusiasts."

—WAYNE L. WESTCOTT, PhD, CSCS
Fitness research director, South Shore YMCA, Quincy, Massachusetts

"*FrameWork* teaches you to understand and respect your body in so many ways. The result is a stronger, more resilient you. *FrameWork* is great prevention for your muscles, bones, and joints, and Dr. DiNubile is the master when it comes to keeping you going."

—KEITH HERNANDEZ
NY Mets World Series Championship Team; six-time NL All-Star and NL MVP; color commentator, MSG Network and Fox Sports Net

"The *FrameWork* plan is innovative, comprehensive, and smart. It's something we all need, especially if you want to go the distance. Dr. DiNubile is a true innovator, and it has been an honor to serve with him on such important committees as the President's Council on Physical Fitness and Sports under the exceptional leadership of Governor Schwarzenegger."

—DR. ROBERT GOLDMAN
President emeritus, National Academy of Sports Medicine, and chairman, American Academy of Anti-Aging Medicine

"Dr. Nick's knowledge of the human frame is extraordinary, and his programs and care have kept dancers dancing for many, many years."

—ROY KAISER
Artistic director, Pennsylvania Ballet

"The more wear and tear you have on your body, the more you need the *FrameWork* plan. *FrameWork* breaks it down so you don't have to break down."

—STEVE SABOL
President, NFL Films

"I was quite young when a knee injury changed my life. Dr. Nick helped me then, and he can help you now. *FrameWork* is great prevention at any age."

—DAVID BOREANAZ
Actor, *Angel* and *Buffy the Vampire Slayer*

"*FrameWork* teaches you how to take optimal care of your body so you can enjoy both life and leisure more. For athletes, it's essential for a long, healthy career."

—JAY SIGEL
U.S. PGA and U.S. Amateur golf champion

"Dr. Nick is a great doctor. Not only an excellent surgeon but an understanding, feeling practitioner in all musculoskeletal-related concerns. As he says, since we are living longer, this aspect of health care has surpassed the common cold for frequency of treatment. I am fortunate enough to have had Dr. Nick repair one of my knees. Being a good example of just the kind of extended-wear person Dr. Nick is talking about, now I am even more grateful to get advice from one of the brightest (and nicest) guys in the field on how to keep my frame working for me. I, like a lot of us who have borrowed time from science, can only very strongly recommend his words to anyone and everyone interested in keeping their bones working to their best potential as we gracefully glide, run, skip, bat, pole-vault, hike, or bike into our happiest days."

—WILLIAM HURT
Academy Award–winning actor

"Nick is a leading physician who inspires and empowers his patients to get active to develop their bodies and enjoy their best health. Regardless of your starting point, his smart techniques and practical guidance can help you get to the next level quickly and safely, whether you're new to fitness, need rehab advice, or simply want to improve your fitness or training techniques to live and feel better. He's also a real standout in the orthopaedic field because of his leadership in "surgery as a last resort." Nick's known for teaching prevention; but when he's helping you manage an injury, he'll guide you through a wide range of less costly treatment options so you can recover quickly. A real bonus is his special expertise in fitness programming to help you strengthen your body's "framework," or musculoskeletal structure and functioning, so your body works more closely to how it is designed. The bottom line: Nick's an expert you can trust to train with to improve your body and feel inspired and capable of moving better everyday!"

—BARBARA HARRIS
EVP/Editorial director, Active Lifestyle Group, Weider Publications, publishers of *Shape* and *Fit Pregnancy*

"What a wonderful book! Finally the individual can learn what he or she should do to make fitness a rewarding, lifelong experience. By decreasing the chances of injury while increasing the enjoyment of activity, *FrameWork* addresses the needs of the individual. No one who wants to exercise regularly should be without *FrameWork*."

—BOB ANDERSON
Author of the classic bestseller, *Stretching*

"There is no other physician in the world of exercise who has a better understanding of how to train and repair the human body, for maximum benefit with minimum risk, than Dr. DiNubile."

—ROGER SCHWAB
Owner, Main Line Health and Fitness; author, *Strength of a Woman*; voted one of the nation's best personal trainers

"*FrameWork* will give you the edge. It's smart and effective and covers all the bases when it comes to longevity, durability, and performance."

—JEFFREY MALUMED, MD
U.S. Ski Team physician member

"This easy-to-read book gives you the same practical advice that Dr. DiNubile gives his patients, and it works well for the couch potato, the pro athlete, and everyone in between."

—JEANIE SUBACH, MA, RD, LDN
Sports nutrition consultant, Philadelphia Eagles, Philadelphia 76ers, and NovaCare Rehabilitation

"Dr. DiNubile's *FrameWork* provides cutting edge information not only from a health and wellness standpoint but from an athletic performance aspect as well."

—GARY VITTI
Head trainer, LA Lakers

Cover and interior photos by Mitch Mandel

Book design by Susan P. Eugster

Library of Congress Cataloging-in-Publication Data

DiNubile, Nicholas A.
    Framework : your 7-step program for healthy muscles, bones, and joints / Nicholas A. DiNubile,
with William Patrick.
        p.   cm.
    Includes index.
    ISBN-13 978–1–59486–057–7 paperback
    ISBN-10 1–59486–057–2 paperback
    1. Exercise—Physiological aspects.   2. Physical fitness.   3. Musculoskeletal system.   I. Patrick,
William, date.   II. Title.
    RA781.D542   2005
    613.7'1—dc22   2005008166

Distributed to the trade by Holtzbrinck Publishers

2   4   6   8   10   9   7   5   3   1   paperback

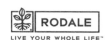

We inspire and enable people to improve their lives and the world around them

For more of our products visit **rodalestore.com** or call 800-848-4735

DEDICATION

■ ■ ■

To those who helped make me a caring doctor:

Connie, Alfred, and Linda

And to those who give me purpose
and keep me striving for excellence each and every day:

Marybeth, Emily, and Dylan

CONTENTS

■ ■ ■

Governor Arnold Schwarzenegger

FRAMEWORK IS A TERRIFIC BOOK by a top-notch doctor dealing with a subject very close to my heart. It's a new philosophy and approach to caring for your body by focusing on the frame.

Over the years, Dr. DiNubile has helped me adapt my own workout to my own, individual frame. He has also helped me when I needed to visit the body shop for repair and rehabilitation. Our friendship began, however, while we worked together on the President's Council on Physical Fitness and Sports during the first Bush Administration, service for which he was honored with the Healthy American Fitness Leaders Award. We continue to work together now with my foundation, After-School All-Stars, a national program committed to helping at-risk inner-city children reach their true potential.

My motto has always been "Stay Hungry," the phrase that was the title of one of my first movies. To me this means never relaxing into the comfort zone, the place where you stop setting and achieving goals. Early on, even though I had many varied dreams, my focus was on building and sculpting the world's greatest body—muscular, but also classically proportioned. Obviously, the gym is where my commitment to that dream was put to the test, but what became clear to me much later is that my focus on exercise was an integral part of every subsequent success. What I did and learned in the gym not only sculpted my body, but also shaped my life. Being fit and making exercise a part of my everyday routine has given me almost unlimited energy. It also instilled in me a determination that carried over into an acting career, the business world, volunteerism, and now, into public service. These habits of mind and body are important for my health, important in facing the challenges of being governor of California, and vitally important in my personal and family life.

As my career has evolved from athletics to entertainment to politics, I have really come to appreciate how the body is a dynamic, ever-changing structure that is different at different times. At 30, you need a different approach to fitness than when you were a

■ ■ ■

teenager. Dr. DiNubile's *FrameWork* offers just that—an individualized program that can be adapted to ever-changing demands and to an ever-changing frame.

The FrameWork Program and philosophy also acknowledges that everyone's body, just like everyone's thumbprint, is unique. This is especially true if you have been as active as I have or if you have had injuries. To achieve my goals early in my career, I had to push my body almost to the breaking point. Clearly, I can't punish my body now the way I did when I was 19. Although I still work out every day, with Dr. DiNubile's help, my regime has evolved along with me.

One thing that hasn't changed over the years is how impressed I am by Dr. DiNubile's passion and creativity. I believe that his FrameWork Program and philosophy is a breath of fresh air, something that will change the way we approach the care and feeding of the human body. I see it as the future of fitness.

No doubt about it, *FrameWork* is an important book that I know you will enjoy and find helpful on your road to optimal health, conditioning, and achievement. It's a must-read for anyone who cares about his or her body and wants it to last. *FrameWork* is just what the doctor ordered.

ACKNOWLEDGMENTS

■ ■ ■

IT WOULD BE ALMOST IMPOSSIBLE to acknowledge the many individuals who have helped influence and shape my thoughts and philosophy as expressed in *FrameWork*. Teachers, patients, and friends—in the gym or on the field—have all had an impact for which I am grateful.

I would also like to extend my sincere gratitude to the following individuals: Arnold Schwarzenegger for his friendship and inspiration over the years, and also "the gang" at Oak Productions—Lynn Marks, Kris Lanin Liang, and Paul Wachter; Lois de la Haba, my agent, who believed in me and in this project from the very beginning; William Patrick for his talent, professionalism, and collaboration; the top-notch, enthusiastic team at Rodale, including Jeremy Katz and Heidi Rodale for their creativity, insight, direction, and support, and also Susan Eugster, Mitch Mandel, Lois Hazel, Deb Cosgrove, Cathy Lee Gruhn, Megan Phillips, Lisa Dolan, and Jennifer Bright Reich; Robert Miller and Kim Strother, whose nearly perfect images grace the pages of this book; Roger Schwab for his friendship, thought-provoking discussions, and state-of-the-art workouts and facility at Main Line Health and Fitness; the Philadelphia 76ers and Pennsylvania Ballet, two first-class organizations I've had the pleasure to work with over the years, and where I have learned firsthand the extraordinary capabilities of the human body—and that given the right circumstances, healing indeed can be accelerated; Jim Teatum at Nautilus; Frank Nein for his help and support in cyberspace, especially at www.drnick.com; my dedicated staff, Mary Moran and Barb DeJesse; and most important, my loving and supportive family—Marybeth, my wife and creative advisor, and my children, Emily and Dylan.

■ ■ ■

PUTTING YOUR FRAME FIRST

THIS BOOK OFFERS the first medically based fitness program for your bones and joints. It's a complete workout, combined with diet and lifestyle advice, designed to address the number one reason Americans visit the doctor—problems with the musculoskeletal frame.

Who's it for?

Elite athletes, complete couch potatoes, and all of you in between.

Seriously.

I don't want to sound like a zealot—or a naïve author—but this is a program for everyone, because everyone with a body needs to exercise. But more to the point, everyone, including—maybe even especially—serious fitness enthusiasts who use their bodies a lot, needs to exercise smarter! The FrameWork way is the only way to make sure you're getting all the benefits of the time you spend working out and that you aren't doing more harm to yourself than good.

Most fitness programs focus on getting you buffed and trim, and, no question, this one is going to help you look great in a swimsuit. But *FrameWork* is not just about looking good. It's also about how you feel and function. It's about durability. It's fitness presented from a medical, healing perspective, the perspective of an orthopaedic surgeon and sports medicine specialist who knows that exercise is a strong medicine. But like any strong medicine, it requires a managed dose.

Your frame is the foundation for every other kind of fitness. Your frame is the anchor for all your muscles, the structural support for all movement. And yet, until now, your bones and joints had to be causing you real trouble before they ever got any attention.

With *FrameWork,* I want to change all that. It's a fitness program designed to give your frame the attention it deserves, building strength and suppleness that will increase your performance, and your enjoyment, of just about everything you do.

The FrameWork Program teaches you to pay attention to what your body tries to tell you about the exercise dosage it needs: when it needs to move, when it needs to rest, what it needs for fuel, and when it's being challenged by a special problem, whether that problem is a heel spur, a bum knee, or stress on the job.

FrameWork offers techniques for building strength and flexibility, for maintaining range of motion, and for stretching, as well as techniques for avoiding reinjury that athletes usually learn from their orthopaedic surgeon, athletic trainer, or physical therapist only *after* they've been hurt.

For couch potatoes, this program is a smart way to get you going without hurting yourself. For athletes and fitness buffs, it's the way to keep going longer and stronger than ever before. For the young, *FrameWork* is the way to learn to exercise right, from the start, to avoid needless wear and tear as well as injury. For anyone over 30, it's the way to work around those dings you've already picked up, to strengthen them, and to make sure you don't reinjure them and put yourself on the sidelines. (In one study of adults involved in a medically supervised fitness program, one-fourth of all exercise participants sustained a musculoskeletal injury. Of these, one-third permanently discontinued their exercise! That is definitely *not* the way to stay fit and healthy.)

Many years ago, as a youngster with faraway dreams of becoming a doctor, I developed a passion for exercise and fitness. When I was around 10, long before bodybuilding had become mainstream, my parents gave me a set of free weights and dumbbells from Sears. I was hooked. I saw something magical about the ability of every individual to sculpt his or her own body. What impressed me then influences me now in how I help others.

But I also learned some lessons the hard way. As a teenager, I shattered my collarbone and missed an entire football season. Several years later, also playing football, I fractured and dislocated my knee. More recently, while horsing around on the beach (as a matter of fact, I was tackled by a well-known fitness guru—you'd think we both would know better by now), I managed to damage a vertebra in my lower back.

So as I work out, I have plenty of weak links I have to work around, which is why it pains me to see people who continue to exercise in a hit-or-miss fashion that invites injury. Others are trapped in the "no-pain, no-gain" mindset that leads to "Fix-Me-Itis," the cycle of injury and repair that qualifies them as the frequent fliers of orthopaedic medicine.

Don't get me wrong—I'm cheering for anyone who makes a commitment to staying in shape. I just hate to see them limping to the sidelines when it doesn't have to be that way. As a doctor as well as a fitness buff, I've learned that you can certainly create problems for your body just as easily in the gym or training room as on the playing field.

I've watched too many runners punish their lower backs and lower extremities. They may have fabulous cardiovascular systems, but too often they have minimal flexibility, which gets them into trouble. Swimmers overdue it with their shoulders. Weight lifters usually overwork their upper bodies and neglect the rest. Golfers and tennis players get back problems and tendinitis.

And I suspect you know some of these people. They're your buddies who can make a social gathering sound like a recovery room, going on about their meniscus tears or rotator cuff problems. Next time you see them, you can tell them for me that most of this damage is entirely predictable—and preventable!

STOP THE MADNESS!

It was this not-so-silent epidemic of injuries and ailments that made me become a spokesman for the American Academy of Orthopaedic Surgeons, working with Cal Ripken and others to try to get out the message that, yes, get moving, but that "no pain, no gain" is not the way to go.

I travel the country to teach physicians about exercise, and I've worked to introduce exercise to medical school curricula. I've also been a special advisor and medical consultant to the President's Council on Physical Fitness and Sports, a member of the Review Panel for the Surgeon General's Report on Physical Activity and Health, and a national medical advisor to Arnold Schwarzenegger's Youth Foundation, After-School All-Stars. I've advised everyone from CEOs, film and recording stars, and political leaders to the Little Leaguers in my hometown. They say I'm one of the most quoted doctors in America—and what they hear me saying, over and over again, is that everyone—from serious runners, to occasional softball players, to the guy or gal who sits at a computer all day—needs to develop the same mindful body awareness that professionals use to stay strong and fit. And like those elite professionals, we need to apply body awareness to normal training and exercise *before* injury occurs.

The FrameWork exercise program actually grew out of my experiences as physician for the Philadelphia 76ers basketball team and the Pennsylvania Ballet, as well as my work with first-tier bodybuilders, including Arnold Schwarzenegger. These professionals almost always have some kind of ding brought on by all their hours of strenuous training: a weak ankle, a problem knee, a sore shoulder. (If you're old enough to vote, chances are you do, too.)

But I found ways to adapt their training to the specific stresses they place on their bodies, as well as to their specific points of vulnerability. I developed special exercises, and special ways of doing traditional exercises, to both strengthen problem joints and to make sure those dings, or weak links, don't get reinjured. I also developed ways to uncover what we call "stealth ailments," problem areas lurking in the background just waiting to flare into big trouble.

Over the past 20 years, I've taken the knowledge I've gained from working with elite athletes and applied it to the everyday people who come to me as patients in my private practice. Many have already tried traditional surgery or rehabilitation to no avail. But by carefully evaluating their frames, I can usually find a solution to their problems.

Usually, by "fixing" the way they exercise, I can avoid having to "fix" their joints in the operating room. I mean, a serious cyclist would never go out riding on a bike with an imbalanced wheel or a twisted frame. Doesn't it make even more sense to pay attention to—and correct—the imbalances in your human frame?

FrameWork is all about following through on the "prevention" mindset. That's one of the reasons we all try to exercise and watch what we eat—to prevent disease from catching up with us. A lot of us are aware of the simple things we can do to lower our risk of heart attack or cancer. Shouldn't we apply the same kind of thinking to our bones and joints?

Believe me, professional athletes whose livelihoods depend on being ready to play every day take preventive maintenance very seriously. Lance Armstrong has to give the same attention to his joints that he gives to the gears and sprockets of his bike.

But what really motivates me to spread the FrameWork message is my contact with young athletes. I hate to see athletes putting all that sweat into trying to build six-pack abs when what they're really doing is setting themselves up for disk problems in their lower backs.

I hate to see guys in their teens or twenties conscientiously pumping iron—muscle shirts on, their caps on backward, looking cool—but doing it all wrong. By focusing only on their "mirror muscles" they create huge imbalances that, over time, can destroy their joints. They use too much weight, which, while it may help build bulk, definitely overloads the tendons and other tissues. They get away with it for awhile, but then Mother Nature strikes back.

Like anything else worth doing, exercise is worth doing right. Improper form alone can strain a tendon to the break point. A quick movement, instead of a slow, controlled one, increases force, which doesn't just give you

that "ripped" look; it can literally rip a muscle loose from its moorings.

You have to exercise the entire muscle and its attachments, not just the bulging belly of the muscle, because a chain is only as strong as its weakest link. It doesn't do you any good—in fact, in can do you considerable harm—to have a big strong muscle, while the tendon attaching that muscle to a bone or joint is hanging by a thread. You can actually strengthen one at the expense of the other. Ask any championship bodybuilder who's "blown out" his pec or quad. He will not describe it as fun.

Young women who're really good at yoga or ballet often get into trouble coming to those muscles from the opposite direction. They increase flexibility—usually a great virtue—but they don't increase the strength to go with it, and that means strength across the entire range of motion. They push the limits of their stretches, which feels great—until that joint laxity makes them vulnerable to an injury.

But one of the most troubling things I see is soft bone, especially when I operate on young female athletes to reconstruct their injured knees. To replace injured ligaments through the arthroscope, I need to create anchoring tunnels in the bones. To drill into the bone of a 19-year-old male, I have to use power tools and all my strength. But with too many of the young women, I can simply rotate the drill bit with my fingers and the metal will easily pass through their bones. These hard-driving young women too often make themselves too thin, dangerously lowering their levels of body fat, which then affects their calcium metabolism and gives them bones that are like butter. Instead of banking up bone density for the future, they're overdrawing the account when they're young. They're still in school and already they suffer from early, preclinical stages of osteoporosis.

Part of the problem is that most doctors don't routinely screen for simple indicators of joint wear and tear such as range of motion and flexibility, much less bone density. Truth be told, most doctors don't really know enough about exercise—or bones and joints, for that matter. (When was the last time your doctor got specific about your exercise program and its impact on your frame?)

On the other side of the equation, many personal trainers and coaches, no matter how knowledgeable, often focus on motivational techniques and programs designed for people with perfect frames. Where they run into trouble is with all the rest of us with not-so-perfect frames. Personal trainers and coaches have been a tremendous boost to the fitness industry, helping countless individuals. However, they're in the business of pushing you to perform beyond your comfort zone, and given your particular frame, that may be just the opposite of what you need. It's this area of knowledge overlap between the surgeons/rehabilitation experts and the exercise professionals that has become my special territory and that makes the FrameWork Program unique.

As an exercise prescription, *FrameWork* recognizes that everybody's body is also unique. The managed dose of exercise that will do the most for you—without harming you—needs to be measured out for you alone.

That's why *FrameWork* gives you options you can mix and match, customizing the regime to fit your own very specific needs.

SCREENING

Customizing the program begins with establishing your individual baseline, and that's where my unique self-test comes in. What I'm asking is very simple and can be summarized in one brief question: Are you built to last?

With the Philadelphia 76ers, we set a baseline for individualized care by testing the players before and after each season. We look for muscle tightness and the imbalances in muscular development that can be early indicators of trouble. The idea is to ward off the sprains, strains, and pulls that sideline players, as well as more serious conditions that can mean surgery, or even the end of a career. When trouble has already set up shop, the idea is to continue training and exercising, but in a way that allows them to:

a) "first, do no harm," while

b) fully rehabilitating and strengthening that particular area of weakness and

c) transitioning them safely and in a stepwise manner back into action.

It's this kind of attention that explains, in part, why the pros seem to bounce back and recover much more quickly than the rest of us. (It's also a lot of hard work on their part. When your livelihood depends on doing rehabilitation, you find the time.)

At the Pennsylvania Ballet, I do a complete biomechanical screening for any injured dancers, but I also evaluate well beyond the injury itself. Many ballet programs have me screen all their young dancers before they advance to go *en pointe*. This way, everyone involved—the dancer and her parents, teachers, directors, and doctors—can be aware of any irregularities in her frame. With this knowledge, we can all work together to help her develop the fittest possible frame—a frame that will serve her well throughout her career, and throughout her life—with far less downtime from injury.

This book is divided into three parts. Part I explains why attention to your frame is so important and why this book was written. Part II outlines the 7-Step FrameWork Program that will give you a healthy frame, which is a frame that is built to last. In Part III, I acknowledge that things don't always go right with your frame and that sometimes it needs more attention. I review some of the current approaches as well as futuristic treatments that will keep you going.

The FrameWork Program begins with Step 1, the self-test. This test allows you to regain control of that sculpting process that's been going on all of your life, whether it's from throwing a baseball or playing the guitar, running track or sitting for hours at a computer, lifting weights or falling out of a tree. For sure, we've all lost the Gumby-like flexibility we may have had as little kids.

The self-test reveals the secrets of your own, distinctive architecture, as well as your own distinctive points of vulnerability. In Chapter 4, where I demonstrate the proper way to do the exercises, I give unique sidebar recommendations linked to these common conditions. I call them OrthoChecks. This al-

lows anyone with weak links or structural ailments to modify the basic workout to maximize the benefit, while minimizing the risk of injury. The result will be a stronger, more fit, more durable you, ready to work and play hard for the long haul.

Every aspect of this program will alert you to signs of more serious conditions and show you how to sort them out from the minor aches and pains that afflict us all. No one should ever play through the pain or settle for rest and ibuprofen, then discover that he has an ailment that needs serious attention.

For the more serious athlete/fitness enthusiast, I'll show how the FrameWork regime can integrate with and amplify your current exercise routine. (Look for "more advanced" versions of the exercises in Chapter 4.) The more advanced you are in your sport or exercise, the more even slight frays in soft tissue, or imbalances in musculature or gait, can lead to injury or sub-optimal performance. It's like a wheel out of alignment on a racecar, as opposed to a wheel out of alignment on a minivan. The minivan might toddle along to the grocery store and back—not much demand is being placed on it—but the racecar will blow out a tire on the first lap.

What matters most—always—is a balanced approached that pays attention to the underlying medical and exercise physiology that I will explain in the next chapter.

MANAGING YOUR MANAGED CARE

Whenever you work with a doctor, a trainer, or a physical therapist, *FrameWork* prepares you to be an active, not passive, participant.

And inevitably, some of us will at some

point still need to go into the shop to get something fixed. That's why the last section of the book helps you think through the process when "a scar is born."

Making informed choices about surgery is hugely important. But my deeper objective is to change the way we spend billions of dollars in this country fixing things surgically that very easily could be prevented. Most people don't even learn the names for the body parts they're grinding and pounding in their workouts until they experience acute pain or disability. This makes no sense at all, especially when it can cause people lifelong disabilities.

Sadly, the situation with bone and joint health today compares with what general health was like 40 years ago, just before we began to hear about the importance of cutting down on fatty foods, getting regular exercise, and not smoking. We've extended the warranty on the human heart, and people are living longer. We've improved care for skin, and people look better. But it's your frame that gets you where you need to go whenever you need to get there. Without the proper care, your bones and joints can all too easily become the limiting factor in your enjoyment of life.

We all have our own reasons for taking care of our frames and keeping them moving gracefully. At one time I wanted to be a star quarterback. Now, as a working guy with two young kids at home, I focus more on being able to play piggy-back than on playing with the pigskin. You may be a hard-driving college athlete who feels great, or you may be a thirty-something who's started getting lower back pain just sitting at a desk. You may want to keep your bones in shape for running marathons, or you may simply want in ensure that you'll never have to "sit this one out," just when the party is getting good. A healthy, flexible frame is a thing of grace and beauty, whether it's on a running back, or a ballerina, or an executive who knows how to wear a suit.

Only about 10 percent of American adults engage in vigorous activity at least five times a week. About 40 percent never break a sweat. Believe it or not, 23 percent of Americans still smoke! And 20 percent of Americans drink more than they should. All of these affect your general health and, specifically, your frame.

FrameWork aims to make it a lot easier to reverse those statistics of unhealthy behavior. At the same time, it aims to make exercise itself far more effective and efficient, and far less likely to do harm to the very body you're trying to help! *FrameWork* is meant to bring your bones and joints up to speed with the healthy heart and flat stomach we're all looking for, but without the unintended wear and tear.

No matter how stiff or supple, how young or how old you are, the idea is to hang on to what you've got, to improve the way it works and looks, and then to keep it working smoothly and looking great for as long as you live. *FrameWork* is not just about how to enjoy a longer life, but how to enjoy life longer *and more fully.*

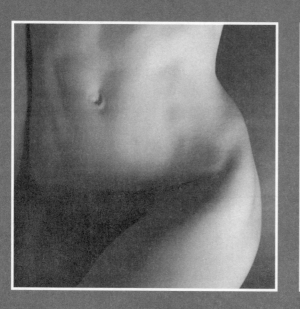
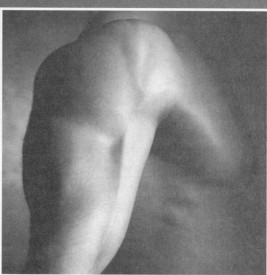

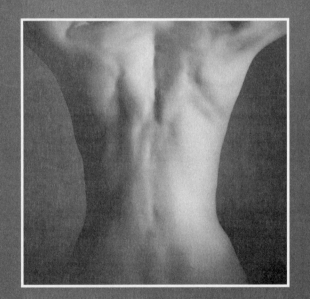

PART ONE

■

WHY

YOU

NEED

FRAMEWORK

ONE

A Different Kind of Fitness

WITH JOSE REYES AT SECOND BASE AND KAZUO MATSUI AT SHORTSTOP, THE NEW York Mets thought they'd acquired baseball's most dynamic duo for the double play. But as spring training for the 2004 season drew to a close, the two young stars had yet to appear together on the same field.

Reyes was out with a pulled hamstring, and Matsui was sidelined with a strained wrist. Having gone 8 years in the Japanese major leagues without missing a game, Matsui, 28, had been considered something of an iron man. But Reyes, only 20, had already become an orthopaedics frequent flier.

During his rookie year, Reyes was benched three times with hamstring trouble, a problem that began for him at age 14. As a youngster back home in the Dominican Republic, Reyes had been running up the stadium steps to strengthen his legs when

he heard something snap. Trouble is, once you pull a hamstring, chances are you will do it again. That's because the muscle heals with scar tissue where healthy cells used to be. Early on in the rehab process, you can reduce the negative effects of that scarring, but it takes a lot of time and a lot of conscientious effort. Once the muscle heals, if you haven't taken full advantage of that window of opportunity, then you get far denser scar tissue with no elasticity. If you look at the muscle under a microscope, instead of the bands lining up parallel and behaving like a spring or bungee cord, the structure is more hap-hazard, which makes it a lot less flexible, and thus more vulnerable—a weak link.

For Reyes, quick, darting movements and sudden lunges are his stock in trade. These movements require sudden contraction of the quadriceps, the muscle in the front of the thigh. This, in turn, requires a quick relaxation and lengthening (eccentric contraction) of the hamstring, the muscle in the back of the thigh. Unless a strong quad is balanced with an equally strong and flexible hamstring, the imbalance is bound to cause trouble.

Whether you play second base or second fiddle, whether you crank miles on the track or code on your computer, you need a frame you can count on. That's why the modern definition of fitness isn't just aerobic capacity, or muscle tone, or the absence of fat. True fitness needs to be from the foundation up, and that means fitness for all the cells and tissues that make up your musculoskeletal frame.

In the old days of baseball, Babe Ruth played until he was 40, but the photographs show an old man with spindly legs and a potbelly, to some extent coasting on his legend. The classic sports novel *North Dallas Forty*, written in the 1970s, portrayed thirty-something pro football players as broken-down old men, hobbling to the stadium, then numbing themselves with painkillers and injections to get through a game. Famous as a great running back before he became infamous as a criminal defendant, O. J. Simpson could be the poster child for this old-school approach to fitness. At his trial for the murder of his wife and her companion, the defense argued that this once great athlete had so many bone and joint injuries, especially to his knees and ankles, that he could barely walk, much less overpower two healthy people! No amount of conditioning is going to fully protect a knee in the National Football League, but today's superstars have redefined conditioning and, as a result, are redefining athletic staying power.

In 2003, *Sports Illustrated* described Oakland Raiders receiver Jerry Rice, then 39, as having "carved up the New York Jets' secondary like a honey-baked ham." In that one game, this "middle-aged man" had nine catches for 183 yards and a touchdown.

That same year, in the National Basketball League, 4 days after turning 40, Michael Jordan scored 43 points in 43 minutes, helping his Washington Wizards defeat the New Jersey Nets, 89–86. He had 10 rebounds, four steals, burst past the opposition to make the game-winning layup, and dived to the floor to save the ball after making a first-quarter steal.

When iron man pitcher Nolan Ryan threw his seventh no-hitter at age 44, and Cal Ripken hung in for 2,632 consecutive games, they were pioneers in terms of durability. But as of 2003, major league baseball had 11 players over 40. As the 2004 baseball season began, Roger Clemens, 41, was still throwing a 96 mph fastball. And on May 17, 2004, Randy Johnson (age 41) warmed the hearts of aging jocks everywhere by pitching a perfect game against the Atlanta Braves, sending 27 youngsters back to the bench without a single hit. In his next outing, against the Florida Marlins, "the Big Unit," as Johnson is called, continued his streak for three more innings before giving up a hit, making a total of 39 batters retired in a row—two short of the major league record. Not bad for an old guy.

Track and field has Regina Jacobs, who at age 40 broke the world indoor record for 1,500 meters. Golf has Jay Haas, who in the spring of 2004—at age 50—was playing so well that some had him pegged to win the Masters. Hockey has Mario Lemieux, who came out of retirement, overcoming cancer and chronic back problems, to captain the Pittsburgh Penguins at age 37. And tennis has Martina Navratilova, who in 2003, at age 46, became the oldest player to win a cham-

■ ■ ■ ■ SIDELINED BY A FAULTY FRAME

Former basketball great Shea Ralph could be the poster girl for the epidemic of knee injuries among female athletes. She's also living proof that no matter how much talent and heart you bring to the game, it doesn't get the job done if your frame gives out on you.

This tall blonde from North Carolina was a dream player with a brilliant future in women's basketball. In 1995–96, she was *USA Today's* "High School Player of the Year." In 1996–97, she was "Freshman of the Year" in *Sporting News* and "Big East Conference Rookie of the Year." In 2000, she was captain of the University of Connecticut women's basketball team that won the NCAA Championship. In 2000, Shea Ralph was an All-American, as well as MVP of the Final Four.

But when it came time to turn pro, and Ralph was drafted by the WNBA's Utah Starzz, she was never able to play. By the end of her college career, Shea had lost her anterior cruciate ligament (ACL) on both sides. In all, she has had to endure six different knee operations.

Her troubles began in the first round of the 1997 NCAA tournament when a fast break turned into an agonized tear in her right ACL. Three days later she had her first reconstructive surgery.

The following year she was redshirted after reinjuring that same knee during a workout. She had her second ACL surgery in September 1997.

It wasn't until 1998–99 that Ralph had her first collegiate start—she made up for lost time by scoring 36 points against Boston College. But then she missed four games with a sprained medial collateral ligament, again in the right knee.

In 2000, Connecticut won all the marbles, and things were looking good for Ralph's career.

Then, in March, 2001, during the first half of a game against Notre Dame for the Big East Championship, she went in for a layup along the baseline, and the crack could be heard throughout the gym—only this time it was her left knee! Another ACL tear.

Today, Shea Ralph contents herself with being assistant coach of the University of Pittsburgh women's basketball team.

In an interview with the *New York Times,* Ralph said that, for a while, she was so bitter about her injuries that she could not even watch basketball on television. Since that low, she's found ways to bounce back and throw herself into the challenges of coaching. But she admits, "I still miss it. I won't lie to you. I really, really would have loved to play pro." We now know that many ACL tears can be prevented by changing the way you condition your frame.

pionship (mixed doubles) at Wimbledon. In 2004, she became the oldest person to win a *singles* match at Wimbledon!

Part of the reason for this athletic longevity is that these players entered the world of serious athletics at a time when serious conditioning was coming into fashion.

Unfortunately, the benefit still hasn't reached everyone.

Too many great young athletes—University of Connecticut basketball's All-American Shea Ralph is a perfect example—see their dreams shattered for no other reason than a faulty frame.

AVOIDING WEAK LINKS

Torn cartilage in the knee or a stress fracture can harm you, whereas a bruise and a small hematoma (swelling) from a kick will merely hurt. A certain degree of hurt is okay—it's the harm you have to watch out for.

The danger of letting "hurt" continue until it causes harm is that, even when the injury can be "repaired," it often leaves you with a structural flaw, a weak link—like Jose Reyes's scarred hamstring—that makes you vulnerable to further injury.

We all have these vulnerabilities in our frames: structural flaws, some big, some small. Some are obvious and/or symptomatic—others quiet, asymptomatic, lurking beneath the skin, waiting for the right circumstance to rear their ugly heads. Many stay quiet for a lifetime but all have the potential to give you grief.

Weak links come in many varieties and can be from:

- An old injury or ailment that leaves a structural flaw

- Imbalances in musculature or flexibility that put stress on particular joints

- Incomplete rehabilitation of an old or new injury or ailment

- Alignment or anatomy problems

- Genetics

- Tissue changes resulting from aging or other causes

- Your mindset or attitude

- Your program design or exercise technique

Many injuries do not completely rehabilitate, something we call IRS, or incomplete rehabilitation syndrome. It takes a lot of work to get back to 100 percent (or as close as possible) after an injury, and most of us stop around 80 to 85 percent when our bodies think they feel okay (i.e., when the swelling is down and the limp goes away). This is a big mistake. Playing at 80 percent often means reinjury.

Likewise, imbalances in strength, flexibility, or both can be a major setup for bone and joint problems. Most of us are at least a little out of balance, which is why your alignment, genetic makeup, or changes that occur from aging also create vulnerabilities in your frame. The weak links that upset me perhaps the most, and are probably the most preventable, are those we inflict upon ourselves with a negative mindset or poorly designed workouts. The importance of all this is that a chain, or should I say your frame, is only as strong as its weakest link. Find those weak links and toughen them, and you are ready to go the distance.

You have to construct your exercise program to work around, or through, your own, distinctive weak links. By my estimation, 80 percent of the adult population needs some degree of customization of their exercise programs to accommodate their weak links. In the self-test in Chapter 4, I'll help you identify your weak links. Then in the exercise routines, I'll show you how to work around them.

YOUR CHEATIN' BOD

Once again, with any form of exercise, you're sculpting your frame for good or ill. The more you do, the more it pays to do it right and make your exercise specific to your objective. But as we develop weak links, our bodies try to find the easy way out, which does not help the cause.

I once saw the legendary Rudolf Nureyev dance on a night when I could tell that his foot was really bothering him. This was at the Academy of Music in Philadelphia, and after the curtain I went backstage where he asked for my advice. He told me he was worried about a "student of his" who was having trouble with an arthritic great toe—a significant problem for someone who jumps for a living. As we talked further and established a bit of trust, eventually he confessed that the dancer with the toe problem was himself.

Of course, I knew that—I'd been watching him all evening trying to compensate for that painful foot.

A master like Nureyev has a thousand tricks to distract your eye from the problem area, but whenever someone has an injury or imbalance, the body tries to pull off the same magic act. It happens so subtly that usually we're not even aware of it. The body starts cheating a little, and compensating a lot, until all the cheating and compensating create a huge problem.

Dancers who don't have a natural hip turnout, who force their turnout, try to compensate. They rotate the shin around more so that the knee and foot is what is turning out, when the turnout should come at the hip. The knee twist that some use to compensate wreaks havoc. A dancer can rotate her foot around and can drop and destroy her arch and midfoot area, create a bunion, or even damage tendons around the ankle.

The body finds a way, even when you're not conscious of it, and it can happen in almost any sport or fitness activity.

A painful or impinged bone in the foot can throw off your gait, which can throw out your lower back. Loss of range of motion in your shoulder can cause distortion, not just in your golf or tennis swing, but in the musculature all across your upper torso. Favoring your right knee can cause you to sprain your left ankle. It can also cause your right quadriceps to shrink in circumference by an inch or two.

This is why mindfulness in your exercise becomes so important, because all too often, you think you are doing the right thing, but your body is cheating and compensating all of your muscles. When people have had a knee injury or kneecap pain, and they do leg lifts to strengthen the quad muscles, they don't get the benefit because their body cheats, using the hip to lift the leg rather than the important quadriceps muscle.

That's why, in this book, I'll show you modifications to prevent you from cheating your body. For example, if you have knee pain while doing simple leg lifts, I'll teach you the modification called "lock and lifts." For people coming off surgery or kneecap pain, it's a smart, effective way to strengthen the thigh without irritating the kneecap.

Patients come in and say they have been working their legs, and I still find that their thighs have atrophied (gotten smaller and weaker). They're just going through the motions of lifting their legs; they're not being mindful about it. Basically, the hip flexor starts lifting the leg and the thigh muscle can actually be totally relaxed. But when you lock your leg, you make sure that the knee is absolutely rigid before you lift it; once in a while you reach down and feel your leg to know that you are actually getting the muscular contraction and workout you think you're getting. The key is to put some mind behind the muscle.

Here's another example. With shoulder problems, if your rotator cuff is malfunctioning and there's stiffness, when you go to raise your arm, instead of using your shoulder muscles, your body adapts by using your upper trapezius and scapula. It is one of the reasons why people with shoulder pain sometimes will have neck pain, too. The wrong muscles start to overwork. The muscles you need to strengthen are getting weaker, and the neck muscles are getting strained. As a result, you develop two problems rather than solving one.

Similarly, when your back is in spasm or in trouble, your body finds even worse ways to cheat, like tilting or rotating your pelvis. When you try to do some exercises for it, you think you're working your back muscles, but you're actually using your buttocks or hamstring muscles rather than your back extensors.

Also, most of us have a very dominant upper and lower extremity and often, during strength training, without realizing it, one side does more of the work and thus reaps more of the benefit, resulting in an even more dominant side. To avoid letting the stronger arm or leg take the other for a ride, concentration is essential during the lift. Also, occasionally try unilateral workouts and compare results. This is especially important when rehabilitating or strengthening an injured or weaker part where multiple unilateral sets are often required.

You need to learn how to feel the muscle you're working, how to know that it is contracted and staying contracted. Otherwise, you're just going through the motions.

THERE'S NO WAY TO CHEAT THE STRENGTH CURVE

A few years ago, a National Hockey League All-Star and MVP goalie came to me because of a groin pull that had caused him to miss most of three seasons in a row. When I tested him, I discovered that his overall flexibility was good to great. However, his strength curve was not balanced at all. He was very strong when his legs were in close together (adducted), but a large part of being a goalie is being able to jump into a split with your legs out to the side (abducted) to block the puck. Whenever this particular hockey star made that kind of split, he had no strength at all, which made him vulnerable to the groin pulls that were threatening his career.

If you stood in close, the goalie could crush you with his legs, but when I had him spread his legs far apart and asked him to pull them in from this more extreme position, which happens to be essential for goalies, I was able to restrain him with one finger. He simply couldn't generate power when his legs were widely extended. He had done a lot of adductor work (a limited portion of the strength curve), and he was strong in his hips, glutes and upper thighs. But once the legs were out at the extreme, he was vulnerable.

The culprit was his exercise regimen.

I created a program to help the goalie develop more strength across the full range of movement, to give him musculature that was more evenly balanced.

Every muscle has two types of strength. There is concentric strength—the pulling in or "flexing"—and there is eccentric strength—the letting back out or "extending." You need both, and yet they are trained and developed differently.

Every muscle also has a unique strength curve. What this means is that different areas in the range of every muscle are weaker or stronger. When you're trying to do a curl, and your arm is fully extended, trying to initiate the lift, that's a weak area. Once you've engaged the weight, overcome inertia, and are moving past the midrange of the muscle, you tend to do okay. With many muscles the midrange might be a sticking point, the spot where you just can't get through it, and that's where your cheatin' bod takes over.

You lean back on the curl. You use the momentum to throw the weight. Depending on how you train, if you work a muscle isometrically, within a limited range, that muscle gets stronger there and maybe within 10 degrees in either direction. The same happens when you cheat, and suboptimally work a muscle, favoring a certain portion of the strength curve.

When you cheat, you're not working your muscle in a balanced way through its entire strength curve. You get stronger in parts of the range but not in the rest, which can lead to trouble. You're tempted to lift an air conditioner, and you seem strong enough at first, but not all of your muscles are up to the task, which leads to a muscle pull, a ligament or

tendon injury, tendinitis, or a rotator cuff injury. Functional strength, used in everyday life and sports, requires a balanced strength curve in all major muscle groups.

With the goalie, we worked them all, focusing on his deficits or "weak links" by strengthening his groin muscles (hip adductors), especially in the weaker, fully abducted portion of his strength curve, while also focusing on rebuilding eccentric strength. And we made sure he went all the way out slowly, and back in slowly, resisting all the way, and not just letting the weights take him in or out. That's how you gain balanced strength.

The goalie had such long legs and good flexibility that we had to do exercises with hand resistance—rubber tubing could have accomplished the same thing—to work his muscles beyond the range of the Nautilus machine. We also did proprioceptive neuromuscular facilitation (PNF) techniques, which use muscle "contract-relax" techniques as well as movement patterns to re-educate muscles by moving them in unusual patterns.

I even had the goalie work with a dancer to show him how to maintain muscular control in these exaggerated positions. Of all athletes, dancers have the most control through the full range of movement, and they are accustomed to working on the extreme edge of their flexibility.

The goalie never missed another game because of a groin pull.

Dancers and goalies differ in the kinds of physical demands they place on their bodies, as do shortstops, equestrians, divers, running backs, pitchers, power forwards, and putters. The same is true for computer jocks, short-order cooks, students, surgeons, stock brokers, and college professors. What they all have in common is the need for a frame they can count on and the desire for a frame that won't give out before they do.

Dancers have a very unusual problem in that so many of them are hypermobile, very flexible people who like to stretch a lot because they're so good at it. I tell them that it's great that you have all this flexibility, but if you don't have strength in that new range that you've opened up, then you are vulnerable. When you're that far out, perhaps beyond the range of your well-balanced strength, all it takes is a bump or jostle, and you can pull a muscle or injure a joint. Dancers do need to be flexible for their craft, but, to prevent injury and for control, they really should have strength throughout their whole range.

EXERCISE INEQUALITY

Not all exercise is created equal (and "I'm on my feet all day" does not count as exercise), which is why a construction laborer or a roughneck on an oil rig is at great risk. They're doing heavy labor every day, fully exposed to the elements, with no time for repair and rejuvenation.

Unlike bone-crushing physical labor that tears you down, exercise programs that build you up are based on the principles of overload, specificity, repetition, rest, and reversibility.

Overload means that a certain level of stimulus is necessary for adaptation to occur.

Specificity of training means that a specific stimulus for adaptation results in very specific structural, metabolic, hormonal, and functional changes in targeted elements of your body. Different regimens have varying results on your skeletal, muscular, or cardiovascular systems.

Repetition means just that—you have to go through the same motions again and again (but not to the point of doing damage).

Rest is an essential step in the building process and without it, gains can turn to losses.

Finally, reversibility means that, if you discontinue training, you may lose the benefits you've gained.

Sorry, folks, but once again we come back to that unpleasant truth: Use it or lose it, which we will expand to "use it right or lose it." Doing any old exercise any old way is likely to do as much harm as good. To get the benefit and to avoid the harm, you have to do it correctly.

EXERCISE ERRORS

It's amazing to me how many misconceptions people have about exercise—even people who spend a great deal of time at the gym.

Here are the seven biggest exercise errors I encounter.

1) Always stretch before exercising.

The bit of truth hidden in this bad idea is that stretching is essential. But the classic (erroneous) idea that became popular in the 1970s is that you have to stretch before your workout to prevent injury. The Centers for Disease Control and Prevention did a study not long ago that demonstrated that stretching before activity really provides no protective benefit; in fact, stretching cold is more likely to cause an injury.

The right idea is to slowly work up to a sweat *before* you stretch or do anything else particularly strenuous. If you're a runner, for instance, start out with a walk, then a slow jog until you warm up. If you're a basketball player, do a light shoot-around first.

The reason is that collagen, the tissue that is the main building block of muscles, tendons, ligaments, and joints, is temperature specific. It's more elastic when warm, stiffer when cold. A cold muscle or tendon is more brittle, so stretching is *not* the way to "warm up." (Besides, stretching is far too important to be thought of as just an opening act. It is one of the headliners in the Main Event.)

Warmup increases the temperature within muscles and tendons as a result of enhanced blood flow and greater metabolic activity. Increased intramuscular temperature before stretching enhances the ability of collagen and the myotendinous junction to deform safely. This makes your musculature more flexible and may protect against strains. The warmed muscle contracts more forcefully and relaxes more quickly so that speed and strength are both increased during exercise. As we'll discuss in greater detail later, fatigue predisposes muscle to injury by diminishing its ability to generate force and absorb energy in equal amounts.

Also, many of the areas you'll be working—especially the disks in your back—have limited blood supply. Light aerobic movement prepares the tissues for exercise by generating warmth and increasing the blood flow that brings nourishment. Accelerated breathing properly causes relaxation—a natural stress buster—but it also ensures adequate oxygenation for nourishment and repair.

One of the many virtues of cross-training is the way it encourages blood flow everywhere as it overcomes imbalances. Joint surfaces have no blood supply, which is one reason they have very limited ability to repair themselves. Joint surfaces require synovial fluid for nourishment. Tendons, like those in the rotator cuff of the shoulder, have a very limited blood supply, which makes healing there slow and difficult. Gentle, rhythmic movements such as those in Tai Chi promote blood flow to tendons and synovial fluid into joint surfaces. As we age, our circulation is less efficient, so the need for gentle movement to get the blood flowing is even greater. That's why Tai Chi is so great for the aging frame (as well as young ones).

2) No guts, no glory—so just tough it out.
Allen Iverson recently was voted the second toughest athlete in the world in *USA Today* (Brett Favre of the Green Bay Packers was voted the toughest.) Iverson, a former quarterback, will try to tough it out anytime, no matter what. I worry that he pushes himself too hard, and eventually it will catch up with him. Toughness can look ugly 10 years later—just like in *North Dallas Forty*. You don't want to be so tough that you put yourself on bottles of painkillers or an aluminum walker someday. Or, at least, you've put yourself out of the game before your time. Will Iverson be playing in his forties? We'll see. Kareem Abdul-Jabbar was tough, too, but he knew how to take care of himself, doing his yoga long before it was the popular thing to do.

I think the real mark of a tough competitor is not just a willingness to take punishment but a willingness to put in the hours of training, year round. It's doing those MedX lumbar exercises in the off-season if you have had low back problems that limit you during the season. A lot of the younger guys think they don't have to do this. They're used to running out on the court and playing.

The older players with staying power all realized they needed to train year round and embraced this discipline early in their careers. I tell the young athletes I see in my practice, most of whom want to skip the training and jump right to the hall of fame, that for every minute Michael Jordan was on the court, he spent at least an hour in the gym or training room conditioning and working out. If you want to "be like Mike," you better do as Mike does—on and off the court.

3) When it comes to weight lifting, it's what you see in the mirror that counts.

Focusing too narrowly on limited objectives can create anatomical imbalances. Millions of guys spend billions of hours doing endless bench presses and curls to build up the "mirror muscles," the ones they see as they work out in front of those mirrored walls in the weight room. This creates an imbalanced tightness in the front of the shoulders, which is just asking for rotator cuff problems.

Too often our exercise routines are like a movie producer who spends all of his budget on the lead actor but forgets to hire a good supporting cast. Everyone seems concerned about their abdominal muscles, for another example, but not enough people pay attention to the back extensors that work in opposition to those abs. That's how you get the guys with six-pack abs and lower back problems.

4) You gotta load on the weight to get results.

The fixation on mirror muscles, along with being too tough for your own good, combine into what I call the "Harley effect." (At the gym where I work out, these guys all have their Harleys parked outside.) A lot of these guys have been pumping iron since they were teenagers; maybe they were jocks in school. It seems to me they spend more of their time demonstrating their strength, throwing the weights around, rather than building strength through slow, steady, and controlled movement. And they're certainly not looking for advice. They think, "Coach showed me how to do this back in 8th grade. I know how to do it. I don't need any help." Trouble is, Coach may not have known what he was talking about. And we've learned a lot about exercise physiology since 1982.

You should never sacrifice proper form for added weight. When you use too much weight, you compensate by "throwing" the bar, relying on momentum, which might impress your friends, but it doesn't do you any good, and it's likely to do you quite a bit of harm.

All movements in weight training, as in stretching, need to be slow, controlled, and steady. Some advanced athletes do drills with sudden, ballistic movement, and there are times when these advanced techniques can be effective. But most of us need to use our gym time for basic strengthening. You build your athletic skills as part of a separate process, usually on the court or playing field.

Good form—and a slow pace—ensures that you achieve the full range of movement, which includes slowly and methodically returning the weight to the resting position. This is vital to exercising the whole muscle to achieve the balanced strength curve. Again, the point of weight training is to work the entire muscle—not just the belly of the muscle—through its full range of motion, both in the concentric (lifting or "positive") phase and in the eccentric (lowering or "negative") phase, to exhaustion, which is when you can no longer do a repetition in good form. Dropping the weight or letting gravity, not your muscles, lower the weight prevents strengthening the important eccentric component of the muscle.

Using less weight, but going twice as slow as most people do, will enable you to sustain load throughout the entire arc of the movement, and it will exhaust your muscle much, much faster. This, after all, is the point of the exercise. That, along with proper rest and recovery between workouts (and nutrition), allows optimal muscle growth.

5) If a little is good, more is better.

Another aspect of the "Harley effect" is that the same Harleys are parked outside the gym almost every day, with the same guys working the same muscles. Unfortunately, when it comes to muscle growth, more is not better. Muscles respond to optimal overload,

then rest. Too much training can cause muscle breakdown and loss. In general, you should never do the same or similar workout two days in a row. This is particularly true of weight lifting and running. However, walking, stretching, yoga, core work, and other lower intensity activities can be done safely every day. In fact, I heartily recommend stretching every day, especially if you are tight jointed or prone to muscle pulls. Also, certain strength-building rehabilitation exercises after injury or surgery should be done daily or even multiple times a day, because here you're not working the muscles to exhaustion, and you actually need more sets and repetitions to stimulate growth and repair in a safe manner.

6) Just do what you love to do.

If all you do is run, you are going to have classic, predictable imbalances. Swimming, biking, yoga—you can pick any activity, and I can tell you what's great about it, but also the risks it poses and the work it leaves undone. That's why there's no perfect, single activity. Each transforms your body differently, and any activity can create imbalances if left unchecked.

Runners who only run will have great hearts, but they will also have extremely tight and overdeveloped calves, relative weakness of the front muscles in the shin area, extremely tight hamstrings, tight lower backs, weak abdominal muscles, wasted upper bodies, and weak quads. Cyclists who only bike have the massive quads, but often an underdeveloped upper body, with tight shoulders, quads, hamstrings, iliotibial band, and hip flexors. Swimmers who only swim have big shoulders and strong backs and generally well-developed legs (especially the upper half, closer to the pelvis), but they will pay a price in their overworked shoulder joints.

Martial arts and ballet come the closest to being the perfect activities, but even dancers and martial artists will have some pretty classic imbalances. Female dancers, for example, tend to work with the knees turned out. We all have a certain rotation in our hips, and people who are born to be dancers have a natural turn out. You can spot a dancer walking a block away. If their feet were the hands on a clock, the time is always 10:10. Their calves are incredibly strong. They have extremely strong hip abductors, but if they don't train to compensate, most have relatively weak hip adductors. And all the work they do *en pointe* or tiptoe (demi-pointe for males), make the overdeveloped calves overly tight.

The trouble with being in too tight a groove with a certain exercise regimen is that, even if you stick with yoga because you love yoga, or weight lifting because you love weight lifting, you're neglecting other areas of weakness, while possibly overinvesting in areas where you're already doing fine.

We'll talk more about this later, but my general advice to all those highly flexible yoginis is to work in some running and some weight training. And, once again, to all you muscle-bound guys pumping iron or crashing the boards in the gym—get down on the mat and start stretching.

7) *Women need to avoid heavier weights to avoid becoming "bulky."*

The average woman, with her very different hormonal makeup than males, almost never has to worry about becoming the Incredible Hulk no matter how much she exercises. The same is true for men whose body type is genetically designed to carry less muscle mass, which is why it's a mistake to ask for training advice from the most heavily muscled guy in the room. It's a little like asking for advice on starting a business from someone who was born rich. Yeah, they might have to work hard, too, but it's different. The guys with huge, rippling muscles, aside from having spent a lot of time pumping iron, are genetically predisposed to have big, bulky muscles. (They also may be less genetically predisposed to injury—so if they do certain lifts improperly and seem to get away with it, don't assume that you can!)

As we discuss in the next chapter, the response of the body to increased load is to lay down extra bone density, along with extra muscle and even build stronger tendons and ligaments and healthier joints. So women especially, even those who do power yoga, need weight training—with adequate loads to stress the muscles—for its bone-strengthening benefits. Bone responds to load. You don't get that response in a pool, or on the stretching mat, or even a stationary bike. It's also very specific. If you walk or run, you build the bones in the hips and legs but not your wrists and elbows. Weight training is the most effective and efficient way to assure that you are strengthening all your bones.

LESSONS FROM THE TRENCHES

What I've learned from bodybuilders—the really great ones—is that there's a lot more to be desired from a workout than just strength or bulk. You need balance.

Aerobic conditioning needs to be a part of any strength program, too. It's the aerobic workout that makes bodybuilders lean, to help create that "ripped" look on stage.

Flexibility is essential; "muscle bound" is not. The guys who walk like robots and seem to have trouble turning their heads are not doing it right.

Progression is a must. The body adapts to load by getting stronger, whether it's in your biceps or in your heart. This means that your program must be adjusted accordingly to continue to reap and sustain maximum results. Gradually increasing the amount of weight you lift or the distance and/or pace of your running, swimming, or cycling is essential. It can also be tricky and the source of major breakdown if not done right, something we'll talk more about, especially in the Active Rest and Recovery section of Chapter 4.

Exercise and rehabilitation need to overlap. When I prescribe exercise for healthy individuals, I draw upon what I know about rehab—in order to *avoid* rehab.

An injured area that is not functioning optimally deserves special treatment—extra warmup and stretching and extra sets with slow pace and moderate load to help rehabilitate the injury. True fitness requires constant attention not just to how your muscles are doing, but also your bones and joints. And perhaps the most overlooked and under-valued aspect of exercise is, in fact, rest and recovery. As we'll discuss in Chapter 4, downtime is an essential part of the body's sculpting process. Rest is when the cells repair and restore themselves from the stress imposed on them by a good workout.

WHAT ABOUT HANDS-ON HELP?

A great personal trainer can be an incredible asset, and there are many dedicated and well-trained people in the field. They've done a great job in activating a segment of the population who otherwise might still be sitting on the sidelines. Beginners can feel uncomfortable and insecure in a gym, and the trainers get them going and keep them motivated.

But estimates say there may be as many as a million individuals offering their services as trainers. A lot of these people are products of weekend courses, and they may not know much more than you do. So when you're picking a trainer, make sure you're working with someone certified through one of the main groups such as the American Council on Exercise, the American College of Sports Medicine, the National Strength and Conditioning Association, and the National Academy of Sports Medicine.

I've seen personal trainers who come in and say, "Here's my program," but that one way means that the work is more about them than it is about you. The routines that have benefited a trainer personally, or those designed for other clients, may not be appropriate for you. You want a trainer who listens as much as he or she talks.

And don't be too impressed just because

someone is an incredible specimen of health and fitness. It's part of their business to look good. They may exercise all day long, every day, and you don't have the time for that. And some trainers may have had a little extra help, either through favorable genes or questionable supplements. So focus on the quality of their programs, their teaching skills, and their ability to motivate you.

A good trainer will test you to measure your current level of fitness and record your body-fat percentages, levels you can lift, and so on. Then the trainer will set reasonable goals for improvement. He or she will be able to modify your program when needed should problems arise—hopefully sooner rather than later.

You want a trainer who is going to take the time to ask about injuries or ailments and who is willing to elicit feedback from you. How do you feel? Does something hurt? Is it just a little muscle soreness or is it joint soreness? And what are your fitness goals, anyway? Again, exercise is not one size fits all. You want somebody who is not only well qualified and certified, but someone willing to individualize the program for you.

FRAME FOCUS

If you lead from your frame, using this FrameWork Program, you can get the whole package: You can lose the fat, condition your cardiovascular system, and achieve the structural integrity that will make you built to last.

The frame is not only fundamental to everything else we do, it's subject to molding forces we may not even be aware of. We can

let those forces do their work outside of our control—until we're limping or shaped like a pretzel—or we can take control and shape our frames to serve our own purposes.

Normal wear and tear is a relative thing. A well-conditioned 60 year old can outperform a poorly conditioned 20 year old—but this is subject entirely to the cooperation (and proper conditioning) of the bones and joints.

Treating your body well retards aging. Not properly conditioning your body, or beating it up through a faulty exercise program, accelerates the aging process. The pace of the aging process is partly determined by genetics, but excessive alcohol consumption, smoking, lack of sleep, and poor nutrition can make you old before your time. The same is true for allowing muscles to weaken or grow imbalanced, for joints to stiffen, and for connective tissues to become brittle.

Running does not cause arthritis in healthy joints. But if you're one of the more than 10 million individuals in this country with some degree of osteoarthritis in your knees, running will indeed accelerate the wear. Ditto for hips and ankles that have early wear.

I see hundreds of patients annually who are in this very predicament. They still feel great when they run, so it's hard for them to understand that they're doing damage to these compromised surfaces. But as I tell them, "You have 10,000 miles left on your knee. Do you want to use them all up this year? Or do you want them to last a lifetime?"

Just as time takes a toll on your skin, it ups

the ante for your frame. Each decade after 25, you lose 4 percent of your muscle mass. After age 40, you lose 1 percent a year. Some people lose more. Unconditioned, you can expect to lose, at roughly the same rate, endurance, flexibility, and the ability to process oxygen. Metabolism also begins to slow in your late twenties, making it much easier to put on weight, which adds to the stress on your bones and joints.

On the happier flip side, vigorous exercise not only retards the loss of muscle, but the muscle you build helps to maintain your more youthful metabolism and appearance.

And it is never too early or too late. William J. Evans, a physiologist at the University of Arkansas for Medical Sciences in Little Rock, did a study proving that even 100 year olds could increase their strength fourfold within a few months through light weight training.

The key is knowing how hard to push yourself and knowing when and how to customize your program. Today we no longer play through the pain, but we pay close attention to the distinction between hurt and harm. That's because, if you want to stay healthy, sitting it out is not an option.

TWO

WORKING WITH WHAT YOU'VE GOT

A FEW YEARS AGO, A GROUP OF SCIENTISTS GOT TOGETHER TO RE-ENGINEER THE human body. They set out to imagine the optimal design for a human frame, meaning a design that wouldn't be so vulnerable to slipped disks, frayed tendons, and worn-out joints.

The "perfect" human design they came up with was short, stocky, and stooped over. It looked nothing like Charlize Theron or Russell Crowe. In fact, it looked like a troll. The upper torso tilted forward, the neck was curved and had much larger vertebrae, the hips were thick with extra muscle and fat, and, strangest of all, the knees never locked but were able to bend backward.

The purpose of this exercise was to illustrate that the human body we rely on has some fundamental flaws built in. Certainly it was never designed to work smoothly for 80 or 90 years. Over most of our history as a species, hardly anybody lived past 40, so what would have been the point of tougher design specs and a more extended warranty?

But the real issue is that nobody ever sat down with a clean sheet of paper to sketch out a perfect design in the first place. The human body we know and love emerged through millions of years of evolution, and evolution is a patch-it-together process that is mostly trial and error. Natural selection simply does what it can with the structures that already exist in the previous generation. It mixes and matches the blueprints (the genes) for these structures, then tests them through competition.

The truly bad ideas die out (fewer offspring survive to carry on the gene), and the ones that work better than the others get passed along through greater reproductive success. Then the selection process sorts through all the possibilities again as the next generation competes for survival, and so it goes. Over many, many generations, the better ideas spread throughout the population, and things generally improve, but only up to a point.

In our case, what nature has come up

with, and what we are stuck with, is a creature with a heavy head, who stands upright, but has a spine that doesn't do well resisting gravity. This results in too much pressure coming down on the vertebrae, especially in the neck and the lower back. (Ever wonder why "Oh, my aching back!" is a modern day mantra?)

In our legs and feet, we have bones that are too thin for the weight we have to bear. And we have many bones that are too thin to withstand breakage. Making matters worse, as we get older, our joints lose their lubrication, our bones lose the minerals that give them stiffness and strength, and our soft tissues lose the suppleness that gives us flexibility.

Over the past few million years, we've upgraded the performance we expect from these bodies of ours, and during the past 100 years, through improved sanitation, better diet, and infinitely better medicines and health care, we've dramatically extended the human life span. But despite this progress, medical science has done nothing at all to improve the basic human frame. We may live to be 95, but without special care, our frame still holds up pretty well for about 30 years. Evolution has not caught up to give you a musculoskeletal system that will last as long as the rest of you.

But even a 20 year old can maintain perfect body weight, run 30 miles a week, eat truckloads of fruits and bran, have thinner thighs in 30 days, and still be a train wreck when it comes to the structural integrity of his musculoskeletal system. Remember Jose Reyes and Shea Ralph, the young superstars on the injured list?

The only way to have a body really built to last—whether you're a major leaguer or a minor lawyer—is to focus on the frame in your exercise and conditioning. If you want to enjoy the whole game of life, including the extra innings modern science offers us, you have to work specifically to offset and overcome the faulty engineering. And that's before you add your own little dings from playing basketball or sitting at a desk all week with slumped shoulders and a craned neck.

Improving the warranty on your frame means changing the way you approach your daily exercise. It's not enough to simply put in the miles running or bang out the hours in the gym. You have to actually think through what you're trying to achieve, then work toward it very mindfully.

Why the FrameWork Program puts the emphasis where it does becomes clearer when you have a better understanding of some very basic anatomy and physiology. I'm going to walk you through some of that right now, and if you come away with nothing else, I hope you'll remember these three things:

1) Bone is dynamic, living tissue. It grows as the body grows, and throughout life it is reshaped, with much of its mass cycled through the system and replaced.

2) Bone is laid down where it is needed, and it is reabsorbed where it is not needed, according to the mechanical demands or stresses placed on it. This is yet another way of saying "use it or lose it."

3) Bone and other structural tissue (like tendons and ligaments) can change shape when overloaded, and the ability to

adapt to increased physical demands depends on timing, genetics, and age. (Which adds the warning label: "Overuse it, or use it mindlessly, and you might lose it still.")

Getting the right balance between exercise that helps and exercise that hurts requires more than bumper-sticker formulations. You have to understand how our bodies are built, and how they respond to the stress of exercise. What are you actually trying to achieve inside your chest muscles when you do a bench press? What's actually happening to your shinbones when you run 10 miles or to your shoulders when you swim 50 laps?

BASIC BONES

The skeleton protects our internal organs; provides a scaffold to support the muscles, skin, organs, blood vessels, and nerves; and gives rigidity and leverage to the muscular action that allows us to move. Because of the way our muscles and bones are joined, and the way the joints that link bones together are articulated, the skeleton is not only rigid, but also flexible.

Bones are also every bit as alive as are the tissues in your muscle or skin (see point #1 on the opposite page). Yes, bones have a high content of inorganic materials, namely minerals, mostly in the form of calcium phosphate, but bones are surrounded by a dense connective tissue membrane, called the periosteum, that contains nerve fibers that pass into the bone cortex. The periosteum also contains blood vessels that keep bone supplied with the oxygen and nutrients it needs.

The organic part of bone consists of millions of living cells, but also a matrix called osteoid, made from a tough, fibrous protein called collagen.

When we are still embryos in the womb, we develop a soft skeleton consisting of cartilage, a highly elastic form of collagen. Later, that rubbery cartilage is invaded by builder cells (called osteoblasts) that replace the soft tissue with new osteoid (the organic matrix) that eventually mineralizes into bone. This process is called ossification.

Even after we're fully grown, though, our bones are constantly being remodeled. They change and renew themselves, replacing obsolete components to preserve structural integrity and prolong normal function. In order to make room for new bone, the old bone—especially bone that has been damaged—is eaten away by cells dedicated to just that purpose. Cells that tear down are called osteoclasts; the cells that build your bones back up are called osteoblasts, and the interplay and balance between the two types of cells is key to your ability to keep on truckin'.

Your hormones, your nutrition, and your level and type of exercise have a direct effect on the balance between building up and tearing down that goes on continuously in your bones.

One of the fundamental rules of orthopaedics is called Wolff's Law, which states that bone is laid down where needed (by way of the osteoblasts) and reabsorbed where not needed (by way of the osteoclasts) in response to the mechanical demands or stresses placed on it. (You may recognize this as point #2 above.)

Wolff's Law is why astronauts who spend a long time in the weightlessness of outer space can barely stand when they return. Their free ride away from the laws of gravity (weightlessness means no heaving lifting) has weakened their bones. Even after a short space flight of 1 or 2 weeks, astronauts, who are amazing athletes in their own right, can lose the same massive amounts of calcium from their bones that elderly patients lose when kept at complete bed rest for 4 to 6 months. On extended space flights of 6 months to a year, astronauts lose not only calcium but up to a fourth of their muscle mass—even with creative in-flight exercise routines designed to combat the zero-gravity environment. A word to the wise: The same thing happens (over a much longer period of time) to people who don't exercise.

SOFT TISSUES

Partnering to give our bodies structural integrity are connective tissues that lack the rigid mineral content of bone. They derive their strength and flexibility from the tough, fibrous, rubbery, and elastic substance we introduced earlier—collagen. While it is a featured player in bone, collagen is a star in the world of soft tissue. It provides not only scaffolding but tensile strength, holding things tightly together, while allowing enough flexibility to move.

We've already mentioned cartilage, the form of collagen that gave us structure before our bones fully mineralized. Cartilage continues to give structure to the nose, ears, and other nonrigid parts of the body. In sports medicine, its most vital role is as a friction

plate to prevent wear and tear on our joints. Cartilage is a smooth, glistening coating for the ends of articulated bones that also provides support, flexibility, and elasticity. It is your joint surface or cushion that, when functioning normally, glides effortlessly as you bend and straighten your joints. With just a single drop of synovial fluid acting as a lubricant, the gliding action of our joints has a coefficient of friction 20 to 30 times that of ice gliding on ice. Now that's what I call a smooth ride.

Articular cartilage does not have a blood supply, so it, along with the chondrocytes (cartilage cells), derives its nourishment from the synovial fluid, a process that is enhanced by movement, especially rhythmic movement like exercise. Motion is lotion. Injured or inflamed joints (synovitis) tend to produce excess synovial fluid, creating a painful swelling with stiffness, as well as loss of strength and motion.

When cartilage becomes damaged, wears thin, or wears out, however, you have the number one medical complaint in the Western World—osteoarthritis. It afflicts almost 30 million (and rapidly rising) people in the United States alone. If you want to have any chance of avoiding this almost inevitable bane of the human condition, you have to start taking care of those bones and joints!

Water accounts for 65 to 80 percent of the wet weight of articular cartilage, and it is this moisture that allows for cartilage to change shape in response to stress, resisting compression. When you squeeze a baby's cheek, or the skin on the back of a child's hand, the skin bounces right back—that's healthy collagen with plenty of moisture. Squeeze the back of an elderly person's hand, and the pressure leaves its mark—a fold of skin that only gradually resumes its shape. Unfortunately this change is not just skin deep. "Drying out" affects your muscles, tendons, ligaments, joint surfaces, and more.

As we get older, collagen also undergoes a process called maturational stabilization, in which the molecules become more tightly bound. Up to a point, this actually enhances connective tissue strength, but in the later part of life, the increasing rigidity of collagen fibers brings stiffness and a greater vulnerability to injury.

Loss of water content in collagen—and therefore in articular cartilage—also affects the disks between the vertebrae in your spine. These shock absorbers should be plump like grapes, but, as they lose water, they become more like raisins.

Drying out reduces flexibility, increases wear and tear, and makes everything more vulnerable to injury. This is why you'll hear me say again and again that you have to drink more water than you ever think you'll need.

In addition to articular cartilage, there's another form called the meniscus, which you start hearing a lot about around, say, your 10th college reunion. Each knee has two menisci, one on the inner (medial) side and one on the outer (lateral) side. Each is a "C" shaped shock absorber for the knee. It also adds to load distribution, stability, and joint lubrication, so when it starts to go, you have problems, and a lot of kvetching about sore knees, torn cartilage, and arthroscopic surgery at cocktail parties.

Another part of the frame's cushioning system is the bursa, a very thin sac formed by two layers of synovial-type tissue located around joints where there is friction between tendon and bone or skin and bone. Examples include prepatellar bursa over the kneecap, trocanteric bursa at the hip, and olecranon bursa behind the elbows. Bursae enhance the gliding of one structure over or across another. When a bursa flares up, it is called bursitis.

Getting Moving

Collagen also takes the form of ligaments—tough, thick, bands that anchor the bones at a joint. Ligaments allow flexibility, but at the same time, they provide stability, binding the parts tightly together. They allow movement, but they resist stretching or bending. Commonly sprained ligaments include the medial collateral ligament (MCL) at the knee and the lateral (outer) ligament complex at the ankle. There is also the epidemic of anterior cruciate ligament (ACL) tears we've described elsewhere.

Ligaments receive their blood supply mainly at the insertion site and harbor mechanoreceptors and free nerve endings that give you awareness of what your body is doing. This contributes to balance. Ligaments also play a major role in stabilizing joints.

Joints that have relatively few or weak ligaments, such as the shoulder, allow greater motion in more directions than joints, such as the sacroiliac, that are virtually surrounded by especially tough and thick ligaments. The bony ends of joints that allow motion are enveloped by a fibrous capsule.

An even thicker type of ligament surrounds and directly reinforces joints such as the hip and shoulder. Ligaments also connect adjoining vertebrae in the spine.

Joints are our hinges, and some, such as the hip or shoulder, allow movement along three planes.

Other joints, such as the elbow, acromioclavicular (AC) joint, or many of the joints in your fingers, allow motion along only one or two planes.

All joints have a definite limit on just how far they can move in any one direction, although some "hypermobile" individuals can bend and straighten some of their joints beyond what is considered normal. Exceed your individual limit and the supporting capsule and ligaments will tear. When it comes to repair and rehabilitation, sometimes a nice clean break in a bone is actually better than a tear. Bones usually heal solid, whereas ligaments often remain loose unless surgically repaired.

Associated with flexibility, but actually quite different, is a concept called joint range of motion (ROM). Flexibility is more about the muscle-tendon unit and its elasticity, or how well it elongates, or stretches. ROM is how much a joint can bend and straighten in its normal arc. We measure ROM in joints like the knee, wrist, or elbow, whereas flexibility relates to muscles like the hamstrings or calves. With arthritis, joint injuries, or surgery, one can lose ROM, but sometimes it creeps up on us without our knowledge. Occasionally these two concepts overlap—your mobility or overall ease of movement often involves both your joint ROM and surrounding muscle-tendon flexibility.

Ligaments hold bones together at the joints, but to power any kind of movement, we need muscle. The collagen structure that connects muscle to bone is called a tendon. We rely on tendons to convey the pulling force of muscle to the bone. They, too, are flexible, but tendons are even less inclined to stretch than ligaments. These tough bands range from the mighty Achilles tendon at the base of the calf to the smaller, more finely tuned tendons that run through the carpal tunnel in the wrist. Limited blood supply in tendons makes nourishment, healing, and repair a problem.

The collagen fibers both in tendons and in ligaments have wavelike, undulating patterns of cells and a matrix called crimp that provides a buffer or shock absorber to protect the tissue during elongation. Then, under loading, the tendon or ligament straightens out and the crimp disappears.

The muscles that primarily concern us in orthopaedics and sports medicine are called skeletal or striated muscles (as opposed to the "smooth muscle" tissue of the heart or gastrointestinal tract). We also call these skeletal muscles voluntary muscle because they are under voluntary control of the central nervous system, powered by the executive suite in the cerebral cortex, otherwise known as your brain. Skeletal muscles are composed of long fibers surrounded by a membranous sheath. It is contractions in the muscle tissue, initiated by an electrical impulse from the nerves that emanate from the spinal cord, that puts things in motion.

Skeletal muscles originate from one bone and insert on another. The bone then functions as a lever. Muscles also act across a joint—or two or more—which then acts as the pivot point or fulcrum. When a muscle contracts, a line of force or pull is created between the two bones to which the muscle is connected.

Many "two joint" muscles, like hamstrings or calves, are much more prone to strain and injury because of this "double-lever" effect.

To produce joint motion, muscles on the side of the motion contract and those on the opposite side of the limb lengthen or relax. (Once again, think of Jose Reyes's quadriceps and hamstrings.) When you need motion in the opposite direction, the lengthened muscles contract and the contracted muscles relax, rotating the joint back to its original position. Joint motion, and consequently body movement, is most often the result of several muscles contracting or relaxing as a coordinated effort.

Again, we come back to balance. Unless you develop your muscles evenly, you can wind up with distortions that will pull your joints out of whack. Without healthy joints, there's not much point in having bigger muscles.

Muscles that produce body movement in the same direction are called agonists, and muscles that produce movement in opposing directions are called antagonists.

A balanced workout makes sure that you work both sets—not just the bicep, for instance, (the agonist) but the triceps (the an-tagonists) as well. Without balance, the tug of war between the two becomes a mismatch.

Just as bone renews itself, so do the cell populations and extracellular matrix of soft tissue. In connective tissues, especially in the musculoskeletal system, there is continual turnover of collagen, primarily in response to tissue loading, both through repeated movement and through the accumulation of load over time.

But just as with bone, either excessive load or prolonged immobilization can trigger a breakdown. Our bodies adapt favorably to graduated increases in physical demand—once again, see point #1—and injury is most likely to occur when we make a sudden change in training. Whenever I treat an athlete with an overuse injury, the first question I ask is about changes in the intensity, duration, or frequency of his program. Even a new or different pair of shoes can be enough to cause trouble.

The lesson from Wolff's Law is that manageable stress on your bones, muscles, and connective tissues is a good thing. But "manageable" is the key word.

To reinforce that idea, we're next going to explore some of the things that can go wrong, then explain how to do things right. An ounce of prevention, after all, is worth a lot more than a plaster cast.

THREE

WHEN BAD THINGS HAPPEN TO GOOD BONES AND JOINTS

THE FORCES YOU GENERATE DURING A WORKOUT CAN AFFECT YOUR BODY PARTS the way a tennis racquet affects a tennis ball. Externally, the force results in acceleration; internally, the effect is momentary deformation. We classify materials as either brittle or ductile depending on the amount of deformation they can undergo before giving out.

Bone is more brittle than connective tissue, and bones are constantly subjected to different kinds of loads. The irregular geometry of bones means that forces come at bone from a variety of odd angles—and sometimes those bones break!

Fortunately, bone heals by regenerating normal bone. There's no scar tissue, and normal strength and function return for young and old alike. The most notable exceptions are among smokers or people whose bones are severely broken in multiple pieces or are part of an open wound. Other musculoskeletal tissues that make up your frame (i.e., tendons, ligaments, muscles, and joints) do not have the regenerative capacity of your bony skeleton, and healing is usually a compromise between regeneration and scar tissue formation. The FrameWork Program is built around the idea that, by exercising right, we can promote optimal repair and regeneration of our frames.

A sudden load that exceeds the ultimate strength of the bone gives you a clean break. But when lower magnitude loads are repeated, usually over prolonged, repetitive physical activity, the result can be a stress fracture. With continued pounding, a stress fracture can become a more traditional complete fracture.

BREAKDOWN

The cartilage on joint surfaces is protected from injury by an embedded network of collagen, proteoglycans, and water, as well as a thin layer of synovial fluid. The underlying

HARD HAT AREA AND STRESS FRACTURES

The remodeling process of bone and other musculoskeletal tissue can resemble a home renovation project. When you want to add on, usually you have to remove existing walls. During the renovation on the way to something bigger and better, you temporarily weaken the structural support. The same thing happens in your body. We know exercise builds stronger bones, but the process begins with osteoclasts tearing down cell walls and removing debris. During this transition period, the body is more vulnerable to injury.

In fact, exercise creates similar transition periods, like the home expansion project, not only in bone but other musculoskeletal tissues like tendons and muscles. The result is a simultaneous building and tearing down, with times of vulnerability, on the way to a stronger, healthier you.

cancellous bone is also able to deform to protect the joint surface cartilage from injury. However, these protective mechanisms may fail and lead to wearing and damage of the articular cartilage. This damage can occur from injury or from abnormal forces produced by poor alignment.

Cartilage can be injured either by a single high-impact load or by multiple, smaller loads that cause an accumulation of damage.

Articular cartilage has little capacity to repair itself following injury because it contains no blood vessels, lymphatics, or nerves. That's one of the reasons why osteoarthritis is the scourge that it is.

Partial-thickness cartilage injuries don't repair themselves either, and sometimes you're better off to have the more serious, full-thickness injury, which triggers the full sequence of inflammation, repair, and remodeling seen in other soft tissues.

We try to protect ligament injuries, often relying on immobilization during the acute (early post-injury) phase, but immobilization has its own problems and can lead to joint stiffness, weakness, and an undernourished articular cartilage, your joint surface. That's why the right kind of exercise, adjusted for your weak links, is usually the better way to go.

In college I tore my medial collateral ligament, a major ligament on the inner side of my knee. I also sustained a dislocation of my patella (kneecap) with a chip fracture as well. I really couldn't walk on my leg, and the orthopaedic surgeon placed me in a long leg cast, which I wore for 10 weeks. At the time, that was considered the correct treatment. Even when I was in training, we used casts for a majority of the walking wounded, but we now know that this may have done more harm than good. Today we favor mobilization or movement whenever possible. When a joint is immobilized, even a normal healthy one, muscles atrophy, the joint stiffens, ligaments, tendons, and other supporting structures lose strength, and even the joint surface loses its protective proteoglycans. The immobilized limb and joint even loses the fine-tuned coordination we call proprioception. Once the cast is removed, it takes a lot of work in rehab to reverse these changes. When muscles and ligaments tear, the type of scar tissue formed is modulated by whether controlled movement or immobilization is chosen. With controlled movement, the scar tissue that forms can be a higher-quality, more durable scar, almost like a natural ligament or tendon. If you look at scar forming in a healing ligament that has been allowed to gently move, the fibers of the scar tissue actually line up in a parallel manner similar to the normal fibers of the tendon. They also behave more elastically and are stronger. The same is true of injured joint surfaces.

Synovitis and bursitis are inflammations of the synovial tissue lining a joint or bursa, often triggered by trauma or overuse. The result is a significant increase in the amount of joint or bursal fluid and the accompanying swelling. Rest, ice, compression, and elevation (RICE) and/or medication usually makes this go away, but sometimes your physician will need to remove it.

Repetitive friction from an overlying tendon or external pressure can trigger bursitis in the shoulder of a weight lifter or pitcher, the elbow of a hockey player or dart thrower, or the knee of a wrestler. If the inflammation is prolonged, the bursae walls may thicken, and sometimes the adjacent tendon degenerates or becomes calcified (calcific bursitis or tendinitis).

Synovitis, or joint inflammation, can be secondary to multiple causes; in the knee, synovitis may result from a meniscal or ligament tear, a contusion, an osteochondral defect (traumatic "pothole" in the joint surface), or a subluxating (loose) patella. In the shoulder, it may follow a rotator cuff injury. Synovitis can also be due to more systemic medical conditions like rheumatoid arthritis, lupus, or Lyme disease.

Joints can become stiff and even freeze up. Conditions like adhesive capsulitis in the shoulder ("frozen shoulder") or arthrofibrosis in the knee are usually caused by an overreaction of the body to injury or overuse. Nerves, too, can be damaged by physical trauma in the form of compression, stretch, or friction caused by anything from weight lifting to computer use. Even long-distance cycling, with your hand held in certain positions for long periods or pressure on your butt from the bike seat, can cause nerve compression injuries. Trauma usually leads to immediate symptoms; symptoms resulting from chronic repetitive or sustained compression may be delayed.

When a nerve glides through a limited space and rubs across a rough structure, various entrapment syndromes can result. Nerves also can be pinched or compressed from spurs or disk herniations in the spinal area, especially the lower back and neck. Abnormal joint motion, such as subluxation (a momentary partial dislocation or shifting out of place because of laxity or instability) may also cause repetitive stretching and injury of nerves that run near the joint. Even poor posture can injure a nerve when you're in tight or unusual positions for long periods of time.

At times, an injured nerve may form a bundle of scar tissue called a neuroma. Neuromas occur after a nerve has been cut or from repetitive trauma or overuse like those seen under the ball of a runner's foot. Tight or poorly fitting shoes can cause a neuroma.

Ladies wearing high heels can develop the same problem.

INJURY: CHRONIC VERSUS ACUTE

There are two major types of injury, chronic and acute. Let's talk about each in turn.

Acute Injury

An acute inury occurs from a sudden, traumatic event, such as a sprained ankle or a fall resulting in a fracture.

Chronic Injury

A chronic injury happens more slowly over time and can be due to old injuries or even overuse-type injuries resulting from repetitive microtrauma rather than one single traumatic event. Remember that joint stress can occur silently, resulting in tissue damage. There is sometimes overlap between acute and chronic injury when a chronic nagging injury has an acute flare-up.

When the injury to soft tissues is chronic rather than acute, protein synthesis can decrease, along with cell division, energy production, storage, and contractility. In addition, the white cells that usually come to the rescue and that clear out debris don't infiltrate as they should. The repair process goes on strike—metabolic shutdown. Even worse, the acute inflammatory response (which is useful in healing and recovery) turns into a more chronic inflammatory cell response (which is not a good thing). The acute, healing cells that are usually "in and out" quickly to clean up the mess of injury become a different cell type that settles in, leads to many chronic painful conditions, and is much harder to get rid of

with treatment. This is one of the many reasons not to let things get into the chronic phase before visiting your doctor.

In the chronic situation, an overall decline in function can occur. This also can result from immobilization, inadequate oxygen supply or nutrition, hormonal deficiency, chronic inflammation, or aging. Atrophied tissues become more vulnerable to sudden dynamic overload or cyclic overloading, which may lead to fatigue and failure, which can lead to injured blood vessels, which can lead to a renewed inflammation-repair process. Once again, that's why, in response to injury, protected activity—the kind of controlled therapeutic exercise I describe in my program—is usually a better treatment than complete rest.

As with bone, the cell populations and extracellular matrix of soft tissues renew themselves. In connective tissues, there is continual turnover of collagen, primarily in response to tissue loading. Here again the body follows Wolff's Law, which states that bone is laid down where needed and reabsorbed where not needed. The trick is to make it work for you rather than against you.

Overuse or overload, combined with cumulative microtrauma, can lead to various forms of chronic inflammation, including lateral epicondylitis, commonly known as tennis elbow.

Tendinitis describes any injury that produces an inflammatory response within the tendon substance. Tendinitis is usually symptomatic, and symptoms may be acute (present for less than 2 weeks), subacute (present for 2 to 6 weeks), or chronic (present longer than 6 weeks). Chronic tendinitis, is usually characterized by both significant tendon degeneration and significant inflammation.

A related condition is tendinosis or tendinopathy, which is actually a degenerative process, most often the result of failed tendon healing seen with aging or repetitive microtrauma. In tendinosis, fibroblasts grow larger, collagen becomes disorganized, and blood vessels are abnormal—all with limited repair capacity. The condition does not usually cause inflammation but can be every bit as painful. Other sites in which we see tendinosis include the Achilles tendon and the rotator cuff. Family history plays a role in such conditions as rotator-cuff complaints, lumbar disk degeneration, and Achilles tendon tears. Certain individuals are at greater risk for connective-tissue breakdown following relatively benign load or use. These athletes may complain of rotator cuff tendinitis, lateral or medial tennis elbow or epicondylitis, and carpal tunnel syndrome, as well as patellar tendinitis, Achilles tendinitis, and plantar fasciitis.

We don't really know what causes this syndrome, but whatever the cause—most likely simply being born with poorer quality collagen—those who are susceptible have to train properly and be aware of their weak links, especially when transitioning to new equipment or new activities.

Chronic overuse is different from acute injury in that it only becomes disabling over time. Vascularized tissues that are exposed to excessive mechanical load wear down, resulting in inflamation. Microtrauma builds up under the radar, until there is the moment of pain or function failure when you know something is wrong.

Because of the often chronic inflammation, accumulation of scar tissue, degenerative change, and atrophy, the recovery from chronic overuse can be slower than the recovery from acute injury. Often, anti-inflammatory measures blunt the pain without doing anything to enhance strength or stability. This, in turn, makes you more vulnerable to reinjury.

SPRAINS AND STRAINS

Some of the most common athletic injuries are muscle strains. These can occur because of inadequate flexibility, inadequate strength or endurance, uncoordinated muscle contraction, insufficient warmup, poor form, or inadequate rehabilitation from previous injury. Sprains and strains are often thought of as interchangeable, but in fact, they're quite different.

A sprain is a stretch or tearing of a ligament. A strain is an injury to a muscle or tendon. Both can be mild, moderate, or severe.

Sprains are categorized as Grade 1 (minimal or slight ligament stretch but overall integrity intact and no joint instability or laxity), Grade 2 (partial ligament tear with elongation of fibers and a mild degree of instability or laxity as a result), and Grade 3 (complete ligament tear with significant instability or laxity). Common ligament injuries include ankle sprains, knee sprains, and finger sprains. The treatment depends on the severity of the sprain and the particular joint or ligament involved and can range from the need for minimal, if any, treatment to the use of a cast or surgery.

Strains are Grade 1 (minor stretch), Grade

2 (more significant stretch with partial tear), and Grade 3 (complete tear or detachment). Common examples include strains of the hamstring, calf, and quadriceps muscles or pec (pectoral) and biceps tendons. Again, as is the case with ligaments, treatment depends on the severity of the strain and the muscle or tendon involved. The most common strains occur when muscle stretching combines with a simultaneous forceful eccentric muscle contraction, especially in those muscles that cross two joints, such as the hamstring or calf muscles. Muscles that cross two joints are subject to greater stretch, and higher forces are possible with eccentric contraction. The mechanical strain occurs when load overcomes the muscle's ability to resist it during deceleration so that the springlike or shockabsorber function of the muscle fails. Muscle strains may be partial or complete, depending on the extent of muscle-tendon unit disruption, but partial tears are more common. Muscle strains produce symptoms such as pain on contraction and stretch, as well as swelling.

I've seen lots of bodybuilders "blow out" biceps and pecs, but the most dramatic muscle injury I ever witnessed happened on the hardwood floor. Charles Barkley, a favorite in Philadelphia before he was traded to Phoenix, and perhaps the greatest power forward ever to play basketball, came down from a jump and fell to the floor grabbing his leg. The huge quadriceps muscle on the front of his thigh, the same one that acrobatically launched him above the rim for many years, had completely detached above his kneecap and rolled up his leg like a shade going up a window. Normal tendons in younger, healthy individuals don't tear during "normal" sports activities, but Charles probably had tendinopathy, a weak link, just waiting to make itself known.

SPORT AND INJURY

As an orthopaedic surgeon, I see many athletes and other active individuals undergoing something akin to premature aging of various body parts based on activities. Each sport has its own unique injury profile. You can predict the injuries and ailments that are most likely to occur, and to the extent that they are predictable, I believe they are preventable.

Basketball players just entering the pros in their early twenties often have ankles that look like they've had arthritis for years. For anybody else we'd say, "Good God! How'd you get that?" But for them, it simply comes with the territory. Basketball players also get patellofemoral wear and defects—areas of joint surface damage where the kneecap rides across the femur, or thigh bone.

Dancers will show degenerative change (osteoarthritis) in their midfoot area, the bones over the arch. In male dancers, as was the case with Nureyev, it's the great toe joint that will prematurely age.

The University of Iowa in Iowa City conducted a test of incoming freshmen football players. At this point, the players' only experience on the field had been in high school, and yet, on x-rays of their cervical spines, over 30 percent showed significant evidence of trauma, including collapsed vertebrae, wedge fractures, spurs, and instability. It's the pounding they do with their heads and helmets that puts them at risk.

While each sport has its own injury profile, each condition can be caused by various factors. Take osteoarthritis as an example. Any sport that involves high-intensity, acute, direct joint impact (football or powerlifting) or both repetitive joint impact and twisting (soccer, baseball pitching) increases the risk of damage, including osteoarthritis. We also know that that high school knee injury puts you at much higher risk for early knee osteoarthritis. Genetic factors account for about half of osteoarthritis in the hands and hips and a smaller percentage in the knees. Otherwise, the cause seems to be a combination of systemic and joint-related factors more than it is one specific serious joint injury.

Early diagnosis, treatment, and complete rehabilitation of these ailments can decrease the risk of greater problems. Simple weight loss can reduce the risk of osteoarthritis, perhaps by half. And strengthening the quadriceps, which is often weak in patients with osteoarthritis, can reduce the risk of osteoarthritis of the knee by 30 percent.

Compounding any damage you might have done to your frame through sports are major changes that happen to our frames as we age. After the age of 40, you lose muscle and bone at about 1 percent per year. In fact, you reach peak bone mass at around age 30 and then it's all downhill. After menopause, the decline for females is even more rapid. Tendons and ligaments lose their elasticity, become more brittle, and tear more easily. The disks or shock absorbers in your spine lose their water content and become less optimal shock absorbers, leading to an increase in neck and lower back problems. Your joints lose proteoglycans and become less durable and start to wear down. The healing process for all these tissues becomes impaired— healing takes longer and is not always complete. You just don't bounce back the way you once did. Metabolic rate slows down, and if you don't increase your exercise or eat less, you gain weight.

But it doesn't have to be such a downhill slide. Many of the changes we used to attribute to added years are actually due to inactivity, not aging per se. They don't necessarily have to happen, as long as you are willing to follow the simple FrameWork Program I lay out in the pages ahead.

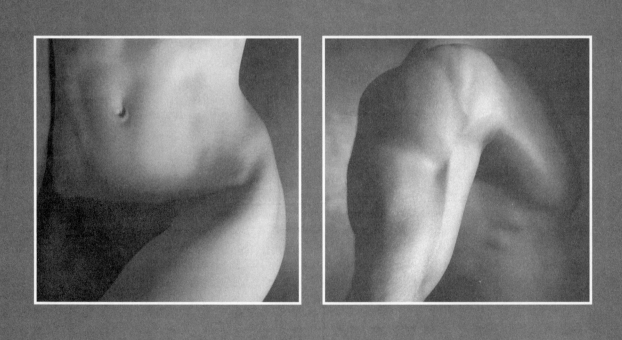

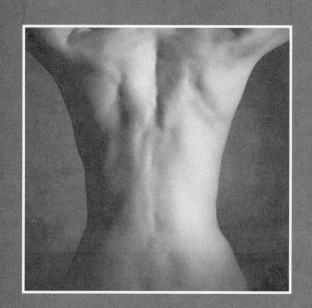

PART TWO

■

THE

FRAMEWORK

PROGRAM

FOUR

THE SEVEN STEPS
OF HIGHLY DURABLE PEOPLE

BECAUSE IT'S SUCH STRONG MEDICINE, EXERCISE DEMANDS CAUTION. IT ALSO deserves your full attention.

The FrameWork Program places your musculoskeletal system front and center, focusing on muscular balance, the oxygenation of tissue, the lubrication of joints, and the application of load so as to strengthen, rather than to compromise or weaken, muscle, soft tissue, and bone.

The physiology I've just explained drives home the importance of proper form and pace, following the logic of a body that is consistently remodeling itself. As I present the exercises, the idea is to work with this remodeling process, not against it.

I present the program in sequence, beginning with slow, simple movement to generate warmth and get blood flowing, thus safely preparing the body's tissues (i.e., muscle, tendons, and joints) for exercise. Stretching, which is different from warmup, comes later. (As I discussed earlier, stretching a cold muscle is an invitation to injury.)

Everywhere, I make a point of proper breathing technique to maximize results. Breathing not only oxygenates tissue, preparing the body for the hard work of exercise, it also improves focus while reducing stress.

But the most fundamental idea for this whole approach is the medical credo *primum non nocere*, Latin for "first do no harm."

With that in mind, let me offer this note of caution: If you've been sedentary, don't launch into a full-scale program of sweat and glory to rebuild yourself into a champion overnight. Instead of dancing around to the *Rocky* theme on the steps of the Philadelphia Museum of Art, you could be in a coronary care unit recovering from a heart attack.

■ ■ ■

ASSESSMENT TOOLS

Before you begin the seven steps of my Frame-Work Program, I strongly encourage you to take this simple readiness test. The Physical Activity Readiness Questionnaire (PARQ) below is an excellent screening tool for seemingly healthy adults who are considering starting an exercise program. The PARQ was developed in Canada to help individuals between the ages of 15 and 69 determine if they need to see a doctor before starting an exercise program. If you're over 69 and not used to being very active, check with your doctor. Anyone answering yes to PARQ question #5, dealing with potential bone and joint issues, should find the FrameWork approach particularly helpful and should always check with their treating physicians or other healthcare professionals before starting a new exercise program or making major changes to their programs.

1. Has your doctor ever said that you have a heart condition and that you should only do physical activity recommended by a doctor?

2. Do you feel pain in your chest when you do physical activity?

3. In the past month, have you had chest pain when you were not doing physical activity?

4. Do you lose your balance because of dizziness or do you ever lose consciousness?

5. Do you have a bone or joint problem (for example, back, knee, or hip) that

could be made worse by a change in your physical activity?

6. Is your doctor currently prescribing drugs (for example, water pills) for your blood pressure or heart condition?

7. Do you know of any other reason why you should not do physical activity?

If you answered yes to one or more questions, talk with your doctor by phone or in person *before* you start becoming much more physically active or *before* you have a fitness appraisal. Tell your doctor about the PARQ and which questions you answered yes. You may be able to do any activity you want—as long as you start slowly and build up gradually. Or you may need to restrict your activities to those that are safe for you. Talk with your doctor about the kinds of activities you wish to participate in and follow his or her advice.

If you answered no honestly to all PARQ questions, you can be reasonably sure that you can start becoming much more physically active. Begin slowly and build up gradually. This is the safest and easiest way to go. It's still recommended that you have your blood pressure evaluated. If your reading is over 140/90, talk with your doctor before you start becoming much more physically active.

The American College of Sports Medicine (ACSM) offers a more comprehensive pre-exercise screening based on your age, health status, current or past symptoms, and medical risk factors. Individuals are then classified either as low, moderate, or high risk to start exercise (See the ACSM Risk Stratification table at right.). Low-risk individuals can usually participate in an exercise program without worry. Those in moderate or high-risk categories usually need a medical evaluation and possible further medical or exercise testing before starting an exercise program.

I recommend that you carefully review both the PARQ and the ACSM guidelines before starting any exercise program. If there is any question about your ability to participate, check with your physician.

ACSM RISK STRATIFICATION*

LOW RISK
Men ≤ 45 years and asymptomatic
Women ≤ 55 years and asymptomatic
with ≤ 1 risk factor *(a)*

MODERATE RISK
Men ≥ 45 years
Women ≥ 55 years,
or have ≥ 2 risk factors *(a)*

HIGH RISK
Individuals with ≥ l sign/symptom of cardiovascular or pulmonary disease *(b)* or known cardiovascular (cardiac, peripheral vascular, or cerebrovascular), pulmonary(obstructive pulmonary disease, asthma, cystic fibrosis), or metabolic (diabetes, thyroid disorder, renal, or liver) disease

   a) Risk factors: family history of heart disease, cigarette smoking, hypertension, hypercholesterolemia, impaired fasting glucose (diabetes), obesity, sedentary lifestyle.
   b) Signs/symptoms of cardiovascular and pulmonary disease: pain, discomfort in chest, neck, jaw, left arm; shortness of breath at rest or with mild exertion; dizziness or syncope; orthopnea or paroxysmal nocturnal dyspnea; ankle edema; tachycardia; intermittent claudication; heart murmur; unusual fatigue, or shortness of breath with mild activity.

* Modified from ACSM's guidelines for exercise testing and prescription.

THE SELF-TEST: ARE YOU BUILT TO LAST?

COMING IN THROUGH THE REVOLVING DOOR, you might think you've stumbled onto a trade show for giants and acrobats, or acrobatic giants. The average height in the hotel lobby is around 6'7"; the average body fat is approaching the vanishing point. The clothing for most of those milling around is Hip Hop casual, with tall lean men wearing brightly colored running suits and baseball caps, and well-developed young women—mostly autograph seekers—wearing not terribly much at all.

This is the June "combines," the annual ritual the National Basketball Association holds in Chicago, just before each year's draft of new players, to allow the teams and their young hopefuls to get a good look at each other.

In addition to the "on-court" evaluation of the players' skills, there are seminars on how not to blow an entire NBA salary on fast cars and "bling bling" and on dealing with the problems of life on the road. The main event, however, is the medical examination. Each of these young athletes must go through an assembly line of physicians, submitting to pokes and probes from perhaps as many as four doctors from each team.

For the orthopaedists like myself, the main thing we're looking for is structural flaws that might lead to trouble down the road. We give the player a good going-over from head to toe, looking for weak links and stealth conditions that might affect his ability to perform night after night, year after year.

If you played sports in school, you probably had some kind of medical exam before you were allowed to compete. With young athletes, doctors are usually concerned about heart murmurs or other systemic conditions that might lead to serious consequences.

But just as we already screen for heart problems, breast cancer, and colon cancer, we need to make some form of musculoskeletal screening a rite of passage for everyone. Pain should not be the only warning light, and injury shouldn't be the first or only call to action. This is why the first step in my seven-step FrameWork Program is a screening self-test that not only detects potential time bombs but also serves as the basis for how to customize the FrameWork Program for you.

The screening program offered here is designed to pick up muscle imbalances; weakness or muscle atrophy; deficits in balance or proprioception (fine-tune joint coordination); loss of range of motion; tightness in back, shoulders, calves, or hamstrings; and, ultimately, design flaws in your past workout, as well as lifestyle issues you might want to consider changing. These are all potential issues that can really mess up your frame if left unchecked.

In addition to helping you make better decisions about your own exercise routine and daily habits, the self-test can help you help your doctor in the detective work of finding signs of wear in your musculoskeletal tissues, the "stealth conditions" that can cause trouble down the road.

The scoring system I devised for *Frame-*

Work follows the scheme my mechanic uses when he goes over my car. Every aspect gets the once over, rated with a check in the box for green, yellow, and red.

Green means smooth sailing.

Yellow means something needs to be watched.

Red means let's do something about it right now.

I've used this color-coded approach for many years with athletes and active individuals in my practice, and I know that it gets us to the heart of the matter very quickly.

As you read through the book, you will understand more about what each item in the test reveals, and why it's significant. These test results also correlate to some degree with the Orthopaedics Top 20 injuries that appear in the Appendix, along with specific modifications for the various exercises in the exercise routines.

If you rated a red light on a past or present kneecap (patellar) problem, for instance, we don't want you doing leg extension exercises the same old way. I'll show you an alternative that will help you avoid further injury while actually strengthening your weak link.

The test is vital to everything that follows, because you can't very well work with what you have—including working around and through your weak links, stealth injuries, and vulnerabilities—unless you know where you are to begin with.

The first items on the self-test are pretty basic to who you are. The list then moves on to lifestyle habits, some of which may not seem relevant at first, various exercise activities, and then specific symptoms. After these simple pencil-and-paper tests, I ask you do to a little moving around to size up how that musculoskeletal system is working.

Take your time taking the test. It not only serves as a screening device, but as a way of learning more about your body. (You also will find an interactive version, with forms you can print out, at the *FrameWork* Web site, www.drnick.com.)

Although the majority of the self-test can be done alone, it is also great to work through this with a partner or even your personal trainer, athletic trainer, or physical therapist. For the problem areas you detect, there are certainly more sophisticated follow-up tests, so you should share your results with your healthcare provider as well as any fitness professionals you're working with.

Caution: These tests may not be easy, but they should be comfortable and not result in any pain. If there is significant discomfort with any of these maneuvers or tests, or if you are unable to perform them, stop that particular test and score a "red." Then check with your physician or other healthcare professional.

The same rules apply here that apply throughout any good workout:

- Slow controlled movements

- No bouncing or ballistic movements

- No forcing beyond comfort

- No pain

- Remember, it's not a competition

THE SELF-TEST: ARE YOU BUILT TO LAST?

LIFESTYLE AND FAMILY HISTORY

Would you say that you're an optimist?

Absolutely	☐ green
Still trying to figure that one out	☒ yellow
What's the point, it all sucks anyway	☐ red

Do you have a family history of knee or hip arthritis?

No	☒ green
Yes	☐ yellow
Knee or hip replacements?	☐ red

Do you have a family history of back problems?

No	☐ green
Yes	☒ yellow
Spinal surgery	☐ red

Do you snore?

Never	☒ green
Sometimes	☐ yellow
Your spouse is ready to toss you out	☐ red

Do you wear out your shoes unevenly, one shoe versus the other?

(Take a pair of well-worn, but not worn out, shoes or sneakers and look from behind at the heel and/or inner arch area. Also look underneath at the wear patterns on the sole, both front and back.)

They're the same	☐ green
Maybe a slight difference	☒ yellow
Very different	☐ red

Do you ever limp?

No	☒ green
Maybe after a hard workout	☐ yellow
Yes	☐ red

Women, have you ever been pregnant?

Never	☒ green
Yes, but no problems	☐ yellow
Yes, and my body has never been the same	☐ red

Did you have any significant musculoskeletal problems (such as knee pain, back pain, sciatica) during or after pregnancy?

No	☐ green
Yes, but it was fully resolved after delivery	☐ yellow
Yes, and it still bothers me	☐ red

How stressed-out are you?

Occasional stress, but I seem to handle it well	☐ green
I feel overwhelmed at times	☒ yellow
Got a Valium?	☐ red

What is your body mass index?

(See chart below to calculate. For a larger view of this chart, see page 157.)

HEIGHT	WEIGHT (IN POUNDS)																			
4'10"	91	96	100	105	110	115	119	124	129	134	138	143	148	153	158	162	167	172	177	181
4'11"	94	99	104	109	114	119	124	128	133	138	143	148	153	158	163	168	173	178	183	188
5'0"	97	102	107	112	118	123	128	133	138	143	148	153	158	163	168	174	179	184	189	194
5'1"	100	106	111	116	122	127	132	137	143	148	153	158	164	169	174	180	185	190	195	201
5'2"	104	109	115	120	126	131	136	142	147	153	158	164	169	175	180	186	191	196	202	207
5'3"	107	113	118	124	130	135	141	146	152	158	163	169	175	180	186	191	197	203	208	214
5'4"	110	116	122	128	134	140	145	151	157	163	169	174	180	186	192	197	204	209	215	221
5'5"	114	120	126	132	138	144	150	156	162	168	174	180	186	192	198	204	210	216	222	228
5'6"	118	124	130	136	142	148	155	161	167	173	179	186	192	198	204	210	216	223	229	235
5'7"	121	127	134	140	146	153	159	166	172	178	185	191	198	204	211	217	223	230	236	242
5'8"	125	131	138	144	151	158	164	171	177	184	190	197	203	210	216	223	230	236	243	249
5'9"	128	135	142	149	155	162	169	176	182	189	196	203	209	216	223	230	236	248	250	257
5'10"	132	139	146	153	160	167	174	181	188	195	202	209	216	222	229	236	243	250	257	264
5'11"	136	143	150	157	165	172	179	186	193	200	208	215	222	229	236	243	250	257	265	272
6'0"	140	147	154	162	169	177	184	191	199	206	213	221	228	235	242	250	258	265	272	279
6'1"	144	151	159	166	174	182	189	197	204	212	219	227	235	242	250	257	265	272	280	288
6'2"	148	155	163	171	179	186	194	202	210	218	225	233	241	249	256	264	272	280	287	295
6'3"	152	160	168	176	184	192	200	208	216	224	232	240	248	256	264	272	279	287	295	303
6'4"	156	164	172	180	189	197	205	213	221	230	238	246	254	263	271	279	287	295	304	312
	19	20	21	22	23	24	25	26	27	28	29	30	31	32	33	34	35	36	37	38

Are you significantly overweight or underweight?

OVERWEIGHT

Good weight BMI below 25	☒ green
Mild overweight 25–29.9	☐ yellow
Higher level overweight and/or obese over 30	☐ red

UNDERWEIGHT

Can't pinch an inch, but there is something there	☐ green
Nothing to pinch, but I can't count my ribs	☒ yellow
Have to run around in the shower to get wet	☐ red

Do you find it harder than 5 years ago to maintain your ideal weight?

No problemo	☒ green
I've added 5 or 10 pounds in the past 5 years	☐ yellow
I've had to have my clothes altered to fit	☐ red

Can you pinch an inch?

No	☒ green
Yes, while sitting	☐ yellow
Yes, standing, too	☐ red

Have you ever smoked?

No	☐ green
Not in the past 10 years	☒ yellow
Got a light?	☐ red

Do you consume more than two glasses of wine (or other alcoholic beverages) a day?

Never	☒ green
Maybe once or twice a month	☐ yellow
Once or twice a week	☐ red

Do you have breakfast?

Religiously	☒ green
Sometimes	☐ yellow
What's breakfast?	☐ red

Is it a healthful breakfast?

With fruit, whole grains, and skim milk or yogurt	☐ green
Coffee and toast	☐ yellow
Coffee and a doughnut	☐ red

What's your daily consumption of fruits and vegetables?

Seven to nine servings and a "rainbow" of colors	☐ green
Maybe a green salad with dinner	☐ yellow
I don't really like vegetables; do fruit loops count?	☐ red

How often to you eat oily, cold-water fish, such as salmon or sardines?

Once or twice a week	☒ green
A couple of times a month	☐ yellow
There's not much fresh fish where I live	☐ red

When you eat on the run, where do you go?

Indian, Thai, Japanese, or Greek	☒ green
Does the salad bar count?	☐ yellow
Would you like fries with that?	☐ red

Do you take an antioxidant supplement that includes vitamins A, C, E, and beta-carotene?

Daily	☐ green
Most of the time	☒ yellow
That's just for health nuts from California	☐ red

Do you take a daily multivitamin?

Daily	☒ green
Most of the time	☐ yellow
I thought vitamins were for kids	☐ red

Do you routinely need to take Advil, Aleve, Motrin, or prescription drugs for muscle, joint, or back discomfort?

No	☐ green
Once or twice a month	☒ yellow
More than twice a month	☐ red

Combining food and supplements, do you routinely consume 1,200 milligrams of calcium every day?

Yes	☐ green
I usually drink some milk and eat some yogurt	☐ yellow
I'm not sure	☒ red

Do you routinely drink sodas?

Never	☒ green
Only the diet stuff, and only now and then	☐ yellow
I'm a colaholic	☐ red

How much water do you take in a day?

8 full glasses	☐ green
4 to 6 glasses, usually	☐ yellow
I'm thirsty now	☐ red

How much do you sleep each night?

6 to 8 hours	☐ green
One hour over or under that span	☐ yellow
A lot more (or a lot less)	☐ red

THE SELF-TEST: ARE YOU BUILT TO LAST?

What is your morning resting heart rate (MRHR)?

(Note: Your pulse rate can be taken either with a portable heart rate monitor or by checking your pulse at the carotid artery on your neck or on the radial artery at your wrist. Do this before getting out of bed in the morning. Count the amount of beats in a 10-second period and then multiply by 6 for your heart rate. When using the carotid artery at your neck, do not press firmly or massage the area because that type of maneuver results in a cardiac reflex that actually slows your heart rate, resulting in a false reading.)

I check my MRHR, especially in times of hard training, and it remains very constant
(i.e., within 5 beats per minute—day to day). ☐ green

I train pretty hard but don't usually check my MRHR, or it's been pretty variable
(i.e., up 5 to 10 beats per minute), and I'm kinda whipped. ☑ yellow

I train very hard but don't check my MRHR, or it's been pretty variable (i.e., up 10 beats per minute). I feel pretty beat, and I'm not making gains. ☐ red

Have you ever taken steroids, growth hormone, or supplements such as androstenedione and DHEA (dehydroepiandrosterone)?

No ☑ green

Yes, in the past (but not in the past 3 years) ☐ yellow

Yes, recent or current use ☐ red

For how many hours at a stretch do you sit at a desk?

Less than 2 ☐ green

2–4 ☐ yellow

More than 4 ☐ red

Are your joints hypermobile?

1. Hyperextend (go beyond straight) your elbows
2. Hyperextend (go beyond straight) your knees
3. Pull your thumb all the way backward to touch your forearm or pull your fingers all the way back so they are at a right angle or beyond to your hand

My joints do not hyperextend. ☐ green

One or more joints slightly hyperextend. ☑ yellow

Call me Gumby! ☐ red

WHAT MAKES YOU SWEAT?

How often do you work out?

Three times a week, an hour a day ☑ green

Maybe once or twice a week ☐ yellow

Let's see, a couple of months ago. . . ☐ red

Does your workout include the following?

Balanced aerobic, strengthening, and stretching	☐ green
A little of this, and a little of that	☐ yellow
Just one thing (running, yoga, swimming, weights)	☒ red

Do you run to get in shape? Or get in shape to run?

I am in shape, or I'll walk, swim, bike (or other low-impact alternatives) till I'm buffed and ready to run.	☐ green
I'll run a little to burn extra calories.	☐ yellow
Running is the best and only way to lose those pounds.	☐ red

For a given sport or activity (bicycling, Rollerblading), do you wear the full protective gear suggested?

Yes	☐ green
Usually	☐ yellow
No	☐ red

Do you stop an activity when you feel pain?

Always	☐ green
Usually	☒ yellow
"No pain, no gain" is my mantra.	☐ red

If you're a runner, how many miles do you log in a week?

Less than 25	☐ green
25 to 30	☐ yellow
30+	☐ red

Do you regularly play soccer, rugby, or basketball, or do you powerlift?

No (or maybe just a little)	☒ green
Once a week at most	☐ yellow
More than once a week	☐ red

INJURIES

Have you had to see a doctor in the past 3 years for any bone, joint, or spine problems?

No	☐ green
One or two visits, no problems now	☒ yellow
Do doctors give frequent-flier miles?	☐ red

Have you ever had an orthopaedic injury severe enough to result in one of the following?

Kept you out of sports or exercise for a month?

Required crutches for 2 or more weeks?

Required surgery?

No	☑ green
Yes (to any of the questions)	☐ red

Have you ever dislocated or separated your shoulder?

No	☑ green
Yes	☐ red

Do you have joint swelling?

No	☑ green
Yes	☐ red

Have you lost mobility (range of motion) in any joint? For example, can you fully straighten (extend) and fully bend (flex)? Compare right to left.

No	☐ green
A little stiff at times but motion is full	☑ yellow
Motion is limited in one or two major joints or spine	☐ red

Do you have stiffness in any joints for any of the following?

Upon awakening (i.e., until showering or moving about 15–20 minutes)

After sitting still more than 30 minutes

For no apparent reason

No	☐ green
Only the day after a hard workout	☐ yellow
Yes	☑ red

Do your knees creak or make noise going up or down stairs?

No	☑ green
Yes, but no discomfort or pain	☐ yellow
Yes, and does cause discomfort and/or pain	☐ red

Do you have trouble actually ascending or descending stairs?

No	☑ green
Only after going up and down multiple times, especially while carrying heavier items	☐ yellow
Yes	☐ red

Does high barometric pressure (i.e., damp, rainy weather) make your joints ache?

No	☑ green
Rarely	☐ yellow
Friends consult me instead of the weatherman.	☐ red

Have you ever had an episode of lower back or neck pain or spasm?

No	☐ green
It kept me off my feet for less than 24 hours.	☑ yellow
I miss work due to recurrent episodes.	☐ red

Do you have pain while lying on either shoulder at night in bed?

No	☐ green
Rarely	☑ yellow
Almost nightly, tossing and turning to get comfy	☐ red

Do you have difficulty falling asleep at night or awaken during the night because of any joint or muscle discomfort?

No	☐ green
Rarely or minor difficulty	☑ yellow
Yes	☐ red

Do you awaken at night with your hands or fingers "asleep"?

No	☐ green
Rarely or I easily shake it off.	☑ yellow
My hand gets more sleep than I do.	☐ red

THE SCREENING TESTS

Is one leg longer than the other?

Tip—ask your tailor or lie facedown—(you'll need a friend to help with this) on a bed with only your feet and ankles hanging off (toes pointing down, legs straight, and feet together). Have your friend look down at your heels (this is sometimes easier to see with shoes or sneakers on). Are the tips of your heels exactly level?

Yes, they are level.	☑ green
Less than 1 centimeter off	☐ yellow
More than 1 centimeter off	☐ red

Foot Arch

Stand barefoot on a hard floor (noncarpeted), with feet shoulder-width apart, feet parallel, and knees slightly bent (and angled slightly in toward each other) like you are skiing. Look at the arch or inner border of your foot and compare to the drawing below.

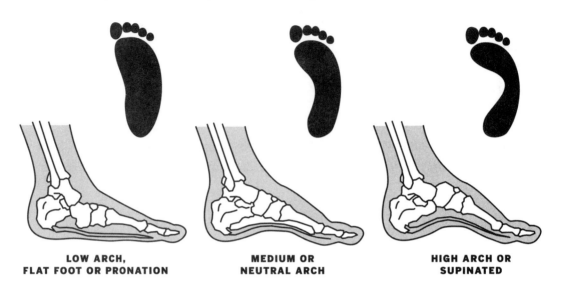

| LOW ARCH, FLAT FOOT OR PRONATION | MEDIUM OR NEUTRAL ARCH | HIGH ARCH OR SUPINATED |

Is the inner edge resting all the way down on the floor (pronation or flat foot) where you could hardly slide a credit card underneath, or is it way up (supination or high arch) where you could slide half a cookie underneath? Or is it somewhere in between?

Better yet, take the "wet test." Dip your bare feet in water. Pat them slightly dry so they are still damp (it may take several tries to get it right). Stand on a large brown bag from the supermarket and make an imprint with your foot. If there is a very large space in the middle where nothing wet touched down to leave an imprint, you have a high arch. Almost no space, low arch. Half and half, medium arch.

Normal arch	☐ green
Slightly high or low	☐ yellow
Very high or very low	☐ red

Ankle Mobility

Stand barefoot with your feet shoulder-width apart, then go down in a slight crouch, like a skier. Keep your heels on the ground. Do both of your knees go equally down and look even and symmetric?

Yes	☐ green
Very close, possible slight difference	☐ yellow
One goes farther forward or one can drop lower without the heel coming off the floor.	☐ red

Knee and Leg Alignment

Stand barefoot, facing a mirror and put your legs together. Look in the mirror. For most of us, our knees will touch slightly, and there may be an inch between your ankles. (A doctor can check this with a standing x-ray of your knee to confirm.) If your knees are touching and your ankles are inches apart, you have a Valgus alignment, you're knock-kneed. If your ankles are together and your knees are apart, you have Varus alignment, or you're bowlegged.

Legs line up pretty straight	☑ green
Ankles together and 1 inch between knees or knees together and up to 2 inches between feet	☐ yellow
Ankles together and more than 1 inch between knees or knees together and more than 2 inches between feet	☐ red

Kneecap Alignment

Stand facing a mirror, feet together, pointing straight ahead.

    Are your kneecaps pointing inward, outward, or straight ahead? Place a dot in the center of the kneecap to help you visualize the path of the kneecap, then picture water squirting straight out from the dots. Is it shooting forward, parallel in the general direction of the feet and toes, or way off inward with the water streams crossing or outward away from your body?

Straight ahead	☑ green
Slightly in or out but still aiming in the same direction as your feet	☑ yellow
Aiming way outward or inward	☐ red

The Stork (Basic Balance)

Stand up straight, extend your arms out wide to your sides, then raise one foot off the ground, up to the level of the opposite knee. Rest the arch of your foot on the inner side of your knee, forming the letter "P." Now close your eyes. How long can you stay balanced that way?

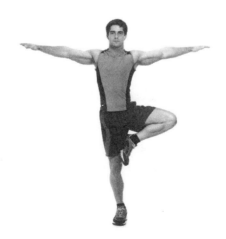

30 seconds   ☐ green
15–30 seconds   ☑ yellow
Less than 15 seconds   ☐ red

Now try the alternate side to see if there is a difference. More advanced balance tests: Try each side but try standing up on the ball of your foot. Next try it standing on a small firm pillow.

The Horse

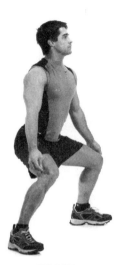

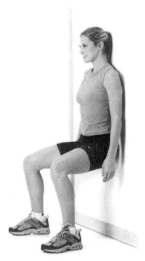

HORSE   **WALL SEAT**

With knees splayed out like you are on a very large horse or small hippo, go into a partial squat (knees bent not quite to 90 degrees). Look straight ahead. If you are unable to do the Horse, try doing the Wall Seat (the easier version until the Horse is possible for you).

Can hold for 30 seconds, then rise easily   ☑ green
Can get down fine, but getting up is hard and/or hold
30 seconds but legs are shakin'   ☐ yellow
Call Jet Li (cause no can do)   ☐ red

Lower-Leg Strength (Hop Test)

Hop on each foot, 20 times right and 20 times left. Note: You should have equal spring with pretty quiet landings. A weak leg would go thud, or your form will begin to deteriorate.

You can go 20 times without weakening.   ☐ green
After 10, your pace becomes a problem or it's uncomfortable.   ☑ yellow
No can do or there's a difference between the right
and left sides.   ☐ red

DO YOU MEASURE UP?

For the next two measurements, you will need either a paper/cloth tape measure or a piece of string or ribbon that can be measured.

Quadriceps (Front Thigh)

Sit on the floor with your legs extended forward and your muscles relaxed. Use a pen to make a mark on the front of your thigh, 4 inches above the upper or proximal edge of your kneecap.

Mark the same exact spot on the other leg, measuring again from the top of the kneecap. Next, measure the circumference of each thigh at that exact level. As you are measuring, gently straighten the leg, while it remains on the ground, tightening the thigh muscle. While measuring, do not pull the tape or string tightly to compress the thigh muscle but just pull it gently to get the exact circumference. Compare the measurements of your legs.

Equal	☑ green
Less than ½-inch difference	☐ yellow
1 inch or more difference	☐ red

Calf Muscle

Sit in a chair and cross your legs. Measure the circumference of your calf at its largest area while relaxed. Repeat for the opposite side. Compare the measurements of your legs.

Equal	☑ green
Less than ¼-inch difference	☐ yellow
¾-inch or more difference	☐ red

■ *Note: If you have upper extremity problem areas, you can measure the circumference of both the upper arm (biceps/triceps) and the forearm, checking for right to left differences. The dominant arm is sometimes slightly bigger, although it shouldn't be if you weight train properly. Also, individuals involved in primarily unilateral sports (tennis player, football quarterback, baseball pitcher) will have greater development of their dominant arms, shoulders, and upper back areas.*

Single-Leg Calf Raise

Stand on one foot with your toes on the first lowest step of a stairway or on a big, stable book. Let your heel drop down so that the heel is lower than the toes by approximately 1 inch at the start of each repetition. Do not "spring" up. Rather, do slow controlled lifts, both up and down. How many calf raises can you do with your left leg, then with your right leg?

20 or more	☐ green
10–20	☐ yellow
Fewer than 10	☑ red

Forearm Flexibility

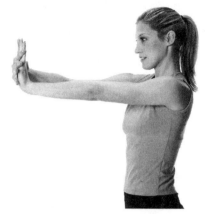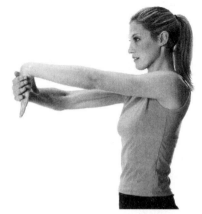

Extend your arms directly in front of you, elbows straight, and hands up like a traffic officer saying "stop." You should be able to make your hands perfectly vertical, your wrists making a 90-degree right angle without any discomfort or strain. Now try the same thing palms down. Again, your wrists should be able to make a 90-degree angle. Can you make a 90-degree angle?

Yes   ☑ green
No   ☐ red

Neck Rotation (Cervical Spine)

Stand sideways to a mirror and look at yourself over your shoulder. Can you turn a full 90 degrees so that your nose is in line with your shoulder?

Yes   ☐ green
Very, very close   ☑ yellow
No   ☐ red

Can you do it with the other side?

Yes   ☐ green
Very, very close   ☑ yellow
No   ☐ red

Neck Flexion (Cervical Spine)

Look straight ahead; now slowly look downward and try to touch your chin to your breast bone. Can you do it?

Chin touches breastbone easily.   ☑ green
Chin is one fingerwidth away from breastbone   ☐ yellow
No way   ☐ red

Neck Extension (Cervical Spine)

Looking in a mirror, touch your forefinger to the tip of your nose and hold it in that exact spot. Then tilt your head back slowly, looking toward the ceiling, to see if you can get your entire chin above the level of your fingertip. Do not lean back; only your head should be moving. Can you do it?

Yes	☐ green
Almost there (i.e., fingertip reaches chin level)	☑ yellow
No way	☐ red

Calf Tightness

Sit on the very edge of a firm wooden chair. With your bare foot flat on the ground, slide your foot back toward the chair slowly, keeping your heel on the floor as long as possible. Looking down, see how far back toward the lead edge of the chair the back of your heel can slide before your heel lifts off the floor. How far back can it go?

Within 1 inch of the lead edge of the chair	☑ green
2–4 inches	☐ yellow
5 or more inches	☐ red

Hip Tightness

Lie on a stable tabletop with your knees and lower legs hanging over the end. Bring both of your knees up until they are clutched to your chest in a "cannonball" position. Now, while one leg remains snug in that position, slowly lower the other. You should be able to place this other knee back fully flat on the table with your leg once again dangling over the side without your other hip coming down or your pelvis rocking forward. If it "hangs up," your hip is too tight. Repeat with alternate leg. How does it go?

Legs go back down fully, easily	☑ green
Legs go back down fully, but feels tight in front	☐ yellow
Leg or legs do not go down fully (i.e., hangs up)	☐ red

Core Strength and Flexibility

Lie down on that same table or on the floor, then tilt your pelvis so that you flatten your back as much as you can while drawing in and tightening your abdominal area. Now, with your legs perfectly straight, slowly raise your heels off the table, then keep going as far as you can without discomfort, ideally until you reach 90 degrees to the hip (feet straight up). How far can you slowly, and in a controlled manner, bring your legs down toward the floor (while keeping them perfectly straight) before you have to arch your back (i.e., no longer able to keep your lower back flattened against the ground)?

Easy up and all the way back down in good form	☐ green
Get 75 to 80 percent down in good form then back area tilts, or it's difficult but able to do without discomfort or back arching	☐ yellow
Can't perform test because of discomfort or lower back tilts early on the way down	☐ red

Core Strength and Endurance (Quadriped)

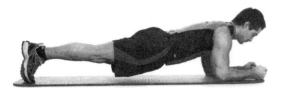

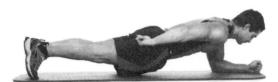

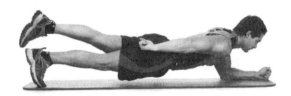

While kneeling on the floor, place your hands flat on the ground as if you were to do a modified pushup. Next, assume the "Chinese pushup" position with your body straight and your full weight supported on both forearms and your toes. Your body should be straight as a board with your pelvis tucked inward, tightening your abdominal and buttock muscles. Try holding that position with your weight on your forearms and toes for 60 seconds. Next, lift your right arm off the ground for 15 seconds, supporting your full weight on your left arm and both feet. Next, return your right forearm back to the ground and raise your left arm for 15 seconds, maintaining proper form. Next, return your left forearm to the ground and raise your right leg for 15 seconds, then return it to the ground and repeat with your left leg. Next, try to elevate your right arm and left leg simultaneously and hold for 15 seconds, then return them back to the ground and try to lift your left arm and right leg simultaneously for 15 seconds. Return to your starting "Chinese pushup" position and hold for an additional 30 seconds. How did you do?

Able to do all positions for the required time ☑ green

Able to do all positions for half of the required time ☐ yellow

Unable to hold all or any positions except briefly ☐ red

Hamstring (Back of Thigh) Tightness

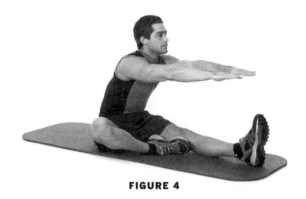

FIGURE 4

Sit on the floor, in the Figure 4 position, left knee straight out with your foot pointing upward and your ankle at a 90-degree angle. Sit tall (as if a string were pulling the top of your head toward the ceiling) and reach forward (like a walking zombie), with your index fingers touching side by side. While staying tall, keeping your chest high, slowly lean forward, keeping your left knee straight, and try to touch the wall (at the level of your eyes, i.e., don't reach down toward toes, but stay tall with good sitting posture). How did you do?

Can place both palms flat on the wall	☑ green
Can reach wall only with your fingertips	☐ yellow
Can't reach the wall	☐ red

Alternate Hamstring Tightness Test

If you have really long arms (and you know who you are), then you might be able to reach the wall even if you have tight hamstrings. Double check with this alternative test.

Lie on your back with your legs out straight. Gently flex the hip of one leg, bringing the knee up toward you until the hip is at 90 degrees with your knee still bent. Keeping the hip at 90 degrees (don't let it drop back down), slowly straighten your knee fully until the leg is out straight and the heel is pointing toward the ceiling. This test is easier to visualize if you lie sideways to a mirror so you can watch your positioning. How did you do?

Leg goes up beyond "L" position with no strain	☑ green
Knee gets almost fully straight but feels tight	☐ yellow
Knee is too tight to fully straighten leg	☐ red

Quadriceps Tightness

Lie on your stomach with your legs extended, knees close together. Keep your knees touching, don't let them drift apart. Then bend your left leg at the knee (or have a friend gently help), bringing your left foot up toward your buttock. Your left heel should be able to touch your buttock while you remain absolutely flat against the floor. If your quadriceps are too tight, either your heel won't *reach your buttock, or you'll have to tilt your pelvis or buttocks area off the floor to accommodate. How did you do?*

Heel reaches buttock easily ☐ green

Can do, but feeling of tightness in front of the thigh ☑ yellow

Heel can't reach buttock or pelvis tilts (lifts up) ☐ red

Shoulder Reach

Reach behind your back with one hand coming over your shoulder, with the other hand reaching up from behind the small of your back. (Try it on both sides.) What can you do?

Clasp my hands ☐ green

Touch my fingertips ☐ yellow *R side tighter*

Are you joking? ☐ red

Shoulder ("Statue of Liberty")

Lie on your back on the floor, with your arms relaxed at your sides. Raise one arm up and over your head with the elbow straight until it comes back down in a full arc toward the floor, like you're doing the backstroke, only with your palm up toward the ceiling in the "Statue of Liberty" position). Repeat with the alternate arm. What can you do?

Shoulder, elbow, wrist all touch the floor ☐ green

Wrist is 2 inches or less off the floor ☐ yellow

Wrist "hangs up" more than 2 inches off the floor ☐ red

Back Rotation

BACK ROTATION

Lie on your back on the floor with your arms full extended out to your sides, palms down. Press your hands against the floor, bring your right knee up and rotate it over your left leg. Without your right elbow, wrist, and shoulder coming off the floor, can you make the right knee do the following?

Touch the floor ☐ green

Come within 2 inches ☑ yellow

Not get within 2 inches ☐ red

■ *Now try it on the opposite side.*

Iliotibial Band (Outer Thigh) Test

Lie on your left side with your legs straight. Now flex your right knee and grab your right foot, bringing your right heel toward your butt. Keeping the rest of your body straight (i.e., your spine, pelvis, and left leg), pull your foot, letting your right knee go back 2 to 3 inches and then allow your right knee to drop back and down behind your left knee, touching the floor. What does your knee do?

Knee easily drops back and down to the floor	☐ green
Knee drops down but is 2 to 3 inches from the floor	☑ yellow
Knee hangs up and does not drop much	☐ red

■ *Now repeat with the opposite side.*

Upper Body Strength—Pushups

Men should do the standard "military style" pushup with only the hands and the toes (not knees) touching the floor. Women have the additional option of using the kneeling or "bent knee" position. (kneel on the floor, hands forward on the floor, keep your back straight). Do as many pushups as possible, without stopping until you can no longer do any in good form. Keep your back straight and let your chest touch the ground on the way down, no bouncing. Count the total number of pushups performed.

MEN	WOMEN	
>25	>18	☐ green
12–25	7–18	☑ yellow
<12	<7	☐ red

Abdominal Strength Crunch-Ups

Lie on the floor with your knees bent, feet flat on the floor, arms crossed on your chest. Pull in and tighten your stomach, push your back flat, and raise high enough for your upper back to slowly come off of the floor. Don't pull with your neck or head and keep your lower back on the floor. How many crunch-ups can you do?

>40	☐ green
25–40	☐ yellow
<25	☐ red

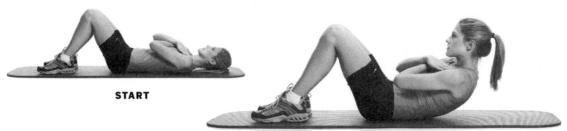

START

FINISH

Posture

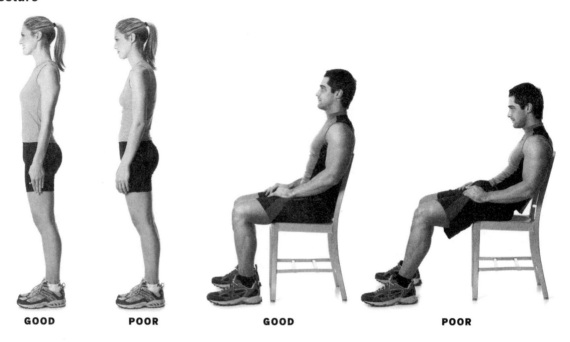

GOOD   POOR   GOOD   POOR

The final item on our self-test is an overall evaluation of how you carry your body—or how your body carries you—and how you present yourself to the world. Get down to a leotard or your underwear and have your partner snap a picture of you from the side standing. (Digital cameras make this sort of thing easy. It is best if the photo is taken when you least expect it, in you natural posture, both standing and sitting.) Then place a ruler over the photograph and draw a line from the back of your ear to your heel. Ideally, the line should bisect your shoulder, pass through your hip, and graze the back of your leg at the knee. How does the picture look?

Straight as a soldier	☐ green
A little stooped	☐ yellow
Playing a hunch	☐ red

Now, take a photo sitting. How does it look and how does it compare with your usual posture?

I sit with good posture most of the day.	☐ green
I slouch only when tired.	☐ yellow
I'm a slouch most of the time.	☐ red

POSTURE TIPS

Stand tall with perfect posture, shoulders back. Have someone place a large strip of 2-inch hypoallergenic J&J or other bandage tape (you can get it at any retail drugstore) across your shoulder blades in your upper back area (like a long name crossing the back of a football jersey). Wear it during the day under your shirt, and you'll feel the pull whenever you stoop or your posture slumps. This little tactile reminder can help you develop new good posture habits, both standing and sitting.

Sit up straight! Flatten your lower back into the chair to ensure that you're neither over-arching nor rounding at your waist. Position your seat so that whatever it is you need to see is directly in front of your eyes. The idea is to not have to tilt your head up or down for an extended period of time. Be especially careful at the computer or when relaxing on a couch or armchair.

Stand up straight! But don't lock your knees when you stand. Bend your knees very slightly to prevent your hips from rolling forward. This takes the pressure off your lower back.

Imagine there's a string attached to your head that's pulling you upward, as if you were a puppet.

Pull your shoulder blades back to square them off so that you could run a straightedge from the back of one shoulder to the other.

When running, hold your head high and look toward the horizon, not down. Don't

▨ ▧ ▩ POSTURE PERFECT

Good posture is not just something they used to teach at "finishing schools." It's the only way to make sure each of your body parts can do its job properly.

Holding onto the proper alignment is a struggle, I admit, because, in almost all of life, the action is in front of us. We lean forward to see, hear, touch, connect. And sitting at a desk or behind the wheel of a car (or on a couch watching TV) only makes it worse. After a while, your shoulders round, your chin goes forward, your lower back collapses, and your belly bulges.

Rather than allowing the spine to do its work, poor posture forces your muscles, tendons, and ligaments to support the body. Over time, these soft tissues begin to conform to this "out-of-shape" shape. Worse, they accept it as the norm and adjust to accommodate. This makes proper form in sports, in dance, and even in walking or running, next to impossible.

A slumping spinal column can't do its job as a shock absorber. The disks between vertebrae are meant to absorb the impact of running or jumping by displacing it through out the spinal column. And when you slump, you can't breathe properly. Shabby posture restricts the flow of blood through the muscles, which means there's less of a "flush" to remove metabolic waste, including lactic acid. So it just pools up in your muscles, increasing the wince factor exponentially, leading to chronic strain of the neck, and upper and lower back.

As we prepare to launch into the FrameWork program, look again at the side view of yourself in the photograph and watch your posture improve even within a few weeks. Most of what it takes to fix these imbalances is just a little concentration during the day.

cross your arms in front of you as you run. This makes your muscles work harder to re-center your torso with every stride.

When resting, lying in the fetal position on a firm mattress is best for your back. Don't tuck a pillow behind your neck; this can crimp your neck. To learn more about how the self-test relates to the health and durability of your frame, see the Appendix, which serves as an index into more detailed discussions in the book about the relevance of each item in the test. It will also refer you to exercise solutions and modifications for problem areas uncovered in the self-test. Or better yet, try the interactive educational version of the FrameWork self-test at www.drnick.com.

With this information about yourself, you should be better prepared to minimize, or even prevent, the wear and tear that wears you down.

My consistent message is that with proper nutrition and a well-managed dose of exercise, you can keep your frame fit, flexible, and ready to go the distance.

The rest of "The Seven Steps of Highly Durable People" will show you how.

HEAVY BREATHING (AEROBIC FITNESS AND OXYGENATION)

WHAT'S THE MOST IMPORTANT muscle in the body?

The heart.

And despite the fact that more than 30 percent of our population is entirely sedentary, plenty of people are getting a good aerobic workout, usually by running, biking, or swimming.

If you're one of them, *FrameWork* wants to complement (and compliment) what you're doing. But beyond the cardiovascular benefit, the aerobic workout in *FrameWork* is designed to provide tissue nourishment and preparedness for the rest of the program. This is why, even if you are an aerobic machine, I recommend that you start your FrameWork workout with a cardiovascular activity to jumpstart the process and prepare your frame for the work to follow.

The fact is, cardiovascular fitness, for reasons that are not entirely clear, actually provides protective benefits for your frame. A landmark study on firefighters, for instance, showed that the ones who were more fit from a cardiovascular standpoint—they weren't necessarily stronger or more flexible—had a much lower incidence of back injuries.

This makes sense, when you consider that movement lubricates your joints and enhances elasticity in your tendons and ligaments. Motion is lotion. If you rest, you rust. And microcirculation is enhanced when you get things moving and your heart pumping. This effect, which also happens with strength training, brings blood cells and oxygen to the nooks and crannies of your body. It also helps clear any "debris" that may be hanging around.

Oxygen is critical at the cellular level for repair, remodeling, and recovery of your tissues—especially in your musculoskeletal system—but there are areas where, day to day, circulation is minimal at best and compromised often. These areas are awakened by rhythmic activity.

So how much of an aerobic workout do you need?

The American College of Sports Medicine's latest recommendation for cardiovascular health is that you need 30 minutes of moderate intensity exercise at least three times a week for cardiovascular health. That isn't a level sufficient for top conditioning—as in, being able to go a quarter in the NBA—but it's the amount of exercise that studies show is necessary to protect your heart from cardiovascular disease and increase your longevity.

Beyond those basics, your need for aerobic conditioning is a question of objectives, as well as certain tradeoffs between helping and hurting, and getting the most benefit for the limited time you have to work out.

By studying groups of individuals over a long period, Stephen Blair, PhD, an epidemiologist at the famous Cooper Clinic in Dallas and the senior editor of the Surgeon General's Report on Physical Activity and Health, has shown that the biggest bang for the buck in aerobic exercise, at least in terms of health protection, is when you go from sedentary to *something*. Sure, there is more benefit when you move from moderate to slightly more intense levels, but it is nothing as dramatic as the rise in benefit that comes with shifting from being a couch potato to simply taking a daily walk or doing a little gardening.

But I did say daily.

A 5-minute walk once a week is probably not going to do you much good, except, perhaps, improving your outlook for those few minutes. But if you can accumulate 30 minutes of moderate activity most days of the week, it's going to be a big plus. You won't be an Olympic athlete, but you'll look and feel better, and you'll be healthier to boot.

Again, the fascinating thing about Dr. Blair's study is that it wasn't just the heart that benefited from moderate exercise. Everything improved, from life span to lower cancer risk.

As a general rule, the best indicator that you're beginning to do something for yourself is breaking a sweat. Even a mild "glow" is good. That warm, slightly looser feeling will happen at different times for different individuals, depending on what shape you're in.

If you've been sedentary, I want you to start with what you're comfortable with. And even before that, I want you to check with your doctor to see what makes sense for you.

If your aerobic exercise is limited to barely breaking a sweat, you're still going to be out of breath when you suddenly have to run up a flight of steps.

For real cardiovascular conditioning, the conventional goal is to attain the range for your target heart rate and maintain that for 30 minutes. In other words, if you want to be truly "in shape," you need to do the following calculation:

1) Take the number 220 and subtract your age. (If you're 30, for instance, that's 220 − 30 = 190.)

2) 190 is your maximum heart rate; you don't want to exercise there!

3) Multiply that number by .60 (190 × .60 = 114) and again by .85 (190 × .85 = 161) to get your aerobic training range.

If you're 30, then, and in good health, your target heart rate is between 114 and 161. To begin a conditioning regime, you need to do some form of exercise that gets your heart rate up to at least the lower end of your training range and sustain that rate of exertion for 30 minutes. And you need to do that three times a week. Then, over time, you work up so that you move toward the higher end of your determined range.

The Borg RPE (Rating of Perceived Exertion) Scale is a very good subjective way to determine how hard your body is working from an aerobic standpoint. It is based on the physical sensations you experience during exercise, including increased heart rate, respiration, and breathing rate, as well as increased sweating and feeling of fatigue. In general, if your perceived exertion rating is between 12 and 14 on the Borg Scale, you are working at a moderate level of intensity. Another way to determine this is to take the "talk test." During aerobic exercise, you should be fairly comfortable carrying on a conversation. You should be breathing harder but able to talk freely. If you are sucking wind and can't get out a sentence, then you are pushing too hard (which may be fine for more advanced training) and are out of the moderate range of intensity.

■ BORG RPE SCALE

RPE SCALE	EQUIVALENT % HR MAX
6	
7 Very, very light	
8	
9 Very light	
10	
11 Fairly light	52–66%
12	
13 Somewhat hard	61–85%
14	
15 Hard	86–91%
16	
17 Very hard	92%
18	
19 Very, very hard	

■

Certain cardiovascular exercises have the potential to stimulate and work the heart more quickly and efficiently. Most people assume that the fittest Olympic athletes are the marathoners, but actually, it's the cross-country skiers and water polo players. Both those activities require the simultaneous use of both upper and lower extremities in a constantly moving rhythmic fashion—a tremendous stimulus for the heart.

If your ability to walk or run is restricted, however, keep in mind that activities that rely exclusively on the upper body can be a powerful stimulus as well. An upper body ergometer (a bicycle that you pedal with your arms) is a great rehab tool to maintain conditioning in athletes who are out of commission with a bum leg or foot. Rowing machines are also very effective and use a good bit of upper body ergometry (in addition to leg and core work).

But while your heart doesn't really care which kind of activity is giving it a workout, your frame very definitely knows. Each activity distributes forces differently across our muscles, joints, tendons, and bones, and sometimes those forces are good and other times not. Your frame will usually tell you—provided that you learn to listen.

It doesn't do much good to have a heart conditioned to run a marathon if your knees are ready for joint replacement.

Doing 60 minutes of aerobic exercise is not twice as good for you as doing 30 minutes. In fact, there's a point of diminishing returns, when the chance of injury, including simple wear and tear, begins to outweigh the gain. When runners go over the 30-mile-a-week mark, running injuries increase exponentially. Ditto for aerobic dance instructors who teach more than 3 classes a week.

Aerobic conditioning is medicinal, and like any other medicine, it has very specific effects and indications for use. A good marathoner can run 26 "5-minute miles," but that doesn't mean that he can run even one "4-minute mile." Because of the way they train, distance runners have enzymes and physiological pathways conditioned for endurance, not speed (though, granted, even a 5-minute mile is still pretty fast).

HOW FIT ARE YOU (FROM A CARDIOVASCULAR STANDPOINT)?
Your heart rate response to exercise is a good indicator of how fit you are. The more fit you are, the harder it is to get your heart pumping rapidly. It is a more efficient pump, and that's also why, with increased cardiovascular fitness,

your everyday, resting heart rate becomes slower.

Your heart rate is a good indicator of overall fitness. Usually the lower your resting heart rate, the more fit you are and the more efficient your heart works as a mechanical pump. A normal heart rate for healthy sedentary individuals is around 72 beats per minute, but as fitness levels improve, this drops into the lower sixties with many elite athletes being well below 60. There are other reasons for a lower heart rate, including certain cardiac problems and the use of certain medications.

Your heart rate can also provide additional information about the inner workings of your body and metabolism. Your morning resting heart rate (MRHR) can be a great indicator of overtraining. Your MRHR should be taken routinely, especially during times of heavier training. It is best taken when you first awaken in the morning before getting out of bed and moving about. You will find, as you get more fit, that your rate tends to be slightly lower, but when you begin to overtrain and overtax your body and its metabolic capability, your

MRHR can begin to rise. An increase in 5 beats per minute can be a warning sign that you are not allowing adequate recovery to your system between workouts. As overtraining occurs, fitness gains drop off and fatigue usually sets in as well as a higher risk of injury. Keep an eye on your MRHR and be sure you are not revving your engine too much.

Fitness can also be measured by how rapidly your ticker slows back down after a bout of heavier exercise. Your recovery heart rate (how quickly your heart rate drops back down after you stop exercising) after strenuous exercise is a good indicator of your cardiovascular fitness, and remember, your overall fitness is a predictor of a more durable frame. However, there is a necessary warning: This test can cause irregular heart beats in people with heart problems, so unless you are in really good shape and are used to higher level aerobic and interval training, check with your doctor before trying it.

To determine your recovery heart rate, check your resting heart rate while sitting quietly and write it down. Next, run in place or do jumping jacks till you break a sweat or your heart is beating fast, and you are at approximately level 15 on the Borg Scale (see page 65). Try to maintain this level for 1 minute. Take your pulse (carotid artery at neck or radial artery at wrist) immediately after stopping and then again 1 minute later and compare.

If your heart does not slow down at least 30 beats in the first minute, you are not in very good shape and are also at increased risk for a heart attack (according to a study in *The New England Journal of Medicine*).

■ ■ ■
CHECKING YOUR HEART RATE (PULSE)

Your pulse rate can be taken either with a heart rate monitor (available at most health clubs) or by checking your pulse at the carotid artery on your neck or on the radial artery at your wrist. Count the amount of beats in a 10-second period then multiply by 6 for your heart rate. When using the carotid artery at your neck, do not press firmly or massage the area because that type of maneuver results in a cardiac reflex that actually slows your heart rate, resulting in a false reading.

This is also sometimes predictive of problems looming on the horizon.

If your recovery heart rate slows down more than 50 beats in the first minute, you're in excellent shape. Also check how many minutes it takes to get back to your original resting heart rate. As you get more fit through the FrameWork plan, you will see your heart rate recovery measure improve.

SPREAD IT AROUND

It's human nature to do what you like to do best during your recreational time; it's also natural to focus where you've developed some skills and where you've established a routine.

But if you're a serious runner, biker, swimmer, hoops player—you name it—I urge you to think about breaking it up and getting more variety into your aerobic workout.

Cross-training really is the smarter way to go. Even if you compete in a particular area, there's much to be gained by bringing in greater balance. Sydney Maree, an Olympic athlete who for a while held the record for the indoor mile, was one of the first distance runners to embrace strength training, even though most runners at that time believed that strength training would "slow them down." That myth was shattered along with many world records as runners and other athletes eventually flocked to the weight room. And if you study the careers of great athletes like Arnold Schwarzenegger, Bruce Lee, Olympic diver Greg Louganis, and wide receivers Willie Gault and Lynn Swann (who integrated ballet into their programs), you'll find lots of examples of getting better at one thing by doing many things.

Many of today's top pro athletes did not play only one sport growing up (like too many of the current crop of young hopefuls). They mixed it up and credit the variety for their overall development as athletes. Each different sport or activity helped develop neuromuscular skills that they were able to apply to their main sports. And there's so much you can do—Tae Bo, dance and martial arts, rope jumping, the elliptical cross-trainer, rowing machines, and the upper body ergometer, to name just a few.

For example, the elliptical machine has been tremendous for individuals with a wide variety of orthopaedic and frame-related issues, especially knee and low back problems, and it remains one of my most recommended cardiovascular workouts. It is very frame-friendly.

The choice needs to be guided by your level, and also the weak links and stealth ailments that showed up in your self-test.

WALKING

Studies show that simply by walking every day, you can reduce your chance of heart attack, stroke, even all-cause morality by 20 to 33 percent!

Walking is one of the safest activities, but even simple walking can have a harmful effect on your frame if you ramp up too quickly, if you pronate, if your arches are too high, or if you don't pick the right shoes.

In studies in which researchers stop people on the street and ask to measure their feet and shoe sizes, a surprisingly significant percentage of people in these random samples are in the wrong-sized shoes. If they like the shoe, and it's even close, they'll squeeze into it.

■ ■ ■
FOOT TYPE

Your foot type can be a risk factor for a wide variety of musculoskeletal ailments from heel pain, shin splints, and Achilles tendinitis to knee and low back problems. The foot bone is indeed connected to the hip bone. Problems can occur at both extremes, high arch (supination) or low rider (pronation). In my experience, most athletes do not know where they stand in terms of arch type. It's important to know not only for injury prevention but also in selecting an appropriate athletic shoe. Pronators will break down the inner border or arch area of their sneakers and need more support in that area as well as motion control. Supinators will often wear out the outer heel area and need more cushioning for shock absorption. In fact, one easy (and free) great way to know your arch type is to ask at a specialty sneaker store that caters to the runners in your area. Also, Road Runner catalog is excellent for helping to decide which sneaker best suits your needs based on not only foot type but also physical demands and body type. Check out the following Web sites for more information: www.brynmawrrunningco.com and www.roadrunnersports.com.

Most people think that your shoe size stays the same once you are fully grown, and that's not always true. Your bones don't grow anymore, but your arch usually collapses and your ligaments relax a little, which adds length to the foot. It's called splay, which means that, especially in the forefoot, things gets wider. When your foot size changes, your footwear needs to change as well. If you were always a seven and you're still buying sevens 20 years later, they may be too tight. That can become an orthopaedic problem, especially if you become an avid walker.

RUNNING

The right footwear is very important for avoiding injury when running is the way you give your heart a workout. That said, running is obviously great exercise. It's simple, it's cheap, you can do it almost anywhere, and it's a great release when you want to shake off all your stressors and cut loose for a while.

But if you run more than 30 miles per week, your likelihood of having some kind of frame trouble goes up. When you run that much, you have to do the cost benefit analysis. The cardiovascular conditioning is great, but what about those knees?

Running on a hard roadway doesn't help. A cinder track or a trail made of bark mulch is better for people with lower extremity issues or those coming off an injury. Running on the beach is a great workout because it demands a lot more; it makes you work harder. But if you have a weak link in your foot, knee, or back, the beach sand will find it.

People like to run barefoot on the beach, and the sand gives in ways that are not always ideal. It's slanted and it's irregular; sometimes it's solid and sometimes it's mushy. So no matter how much you normally run on a straightaway, you should look at beach running as a separate activity and build up to it. Perhaps a walk-jog on your first few days at the beach is the better idea. Even running on a slightly banked roadway can create the same effect as if your legs were different lengths. It causes your pelvis to tilt, and after a certain number of steps, that odd wear is going to have an effect.

As you place one foot in front of the other, the endless repetitions can exaggerate the effect of any small imbalance. If you're a few pounds overweight, that adds stress to the bones in your knees, legs, and ankles. For every extra pound you're carrying, your knees feel the added force of 5 to 7 pounds, which adds up. That's why, if you're overweight, you need to get in shape to run rather than run to get in shape.

And again, you need to have the right shoes. You might even need some sort of orthotic device to straighten out any imbalance. These inserts can be expensive but—if you need them—they can save you enormously.

If you already have a little arthritis in your knee, running is probably not the smartest thing, because you're accelerating wear and tear. I have patients come in who never had a problem until they twisted their knees and tore some cartilage. Their x-rays don't look too bad, but then when I look directly at the joint surface through the arthroscope, I can see all the wear and tear that simply hasn't show up yet on the film or even the MRI. With the injury comes a further loss of cartilage (i.e., torn meniscus), so by now they have lost quite a bit of shock absorption. Add that to the arthritic wear, and you have a knee with only so many more miles on it.

I even tell some of my patients, "You have 10,000 miles left on your knee, do you want to use it all up this year, or do you want it to last a lifetime?" Part of the issue is genetics. Some people are cut out to be marathoners at 80, and other people probably shouldn't be running much past 40. And the fact is, genetics plus injury can put an 80-year-old knee in a 40 year old!

Running does not cause arthritis, per se.

Studies have been done on healthy, elderly distance runners who have no higher incidence of arthritis than the average person. But if you have osteoarthritis, running will surely accelerate it.

You simply have to listen to your body.

CYCLING

Cycling, too, is a great workout, but it raises other safety issues. There are hundreds of thousands of serious injuries on bicycles every year. Usually it's not the bike, it's the roads with potholes, the city streets with car doors opening, and parked cars pulling out.

Regardless of where you ride, you always have to have the proper safety equipment. Most of the serious injuries and death from cycling are head injuries, and a $40 helmet can save your life.

We think of cycling as low impact, and while it causes less wear and tear than running, 1 hour of cycling means, on average, maybe 5,000 pedal revolutions. This means that the smallest amount of misalignment can cause trouble, and cyclists are known to suffer from carpal tunnel syndrome from vibration and positioning, along with neck strain and nerve injuries, not to mention excessive wear in the lower extremities, especially the knee. In a survey done of one long-distance bicycling tour, 65 percent of riders reported knee pain.

Knee injuries, including those most often associated with cycling—anterior knee pain and patellofemoral pain syndrome—are among the most common overuse injuries seen in sports medicine centers.

The repetitive loading causes tissue damage, which eventually tires out a specific structure, such as tendon or bone. Without adequate recovery, the microtrauma stimulates an inflammatory response, which causes the release of inflammatory cells and enzymes that damage local tissue. Continue the microtrauma long enough, and it leads to clinical injury. In cycling, the problems often are not just acute tissue inflammation, but also chronic degeneration—tendinosis rather than tendinitis.

Lack of flexibility also causes problems. Most cyclists' quadriceps and hamstrings will tighten with prolonged riding, and the restricted range of motion around the knee is likely to increase the forces on the knee. Weakness in the leg muscles may lead to fatigue-induced alterations in pedaling technique, which will also alter the forces on the knee. If the seat is the wrong height or improperly aligned, the repetitive forces affecting the knee are even more likely to cause injury.

For women, the increased angle of the thigh bone coming down from the hip may further stress the knee joint during the recovery phase of the pedal stroke.

To get a good cycling workout without problems, then, you have to think not only about your muscle imbalances, your flexibility, your training distance and intensity, but also about that other frame—your bike.

Production bikes are built for averages, yet an ill-fitting bike will leave you tired or, worse, in pain, and you won't be able to climb or accelerate efficiently.

At the very least, the salesperson where you get your bike should measure and adjust the handlebar stem and seat post before and after your test ride. And if you're going to pull your old bike out of the garage and give it a go, first take it down to a local bike shop for a tuneup and safety check. While you're there, check the fit.

The saddle may be too low, too far forward, or both, causing excessive patellofemoral loading throughout the pedal cycle. When the saddle is low, the knee functions in hyperflexion, increasing compression of the patella on the femur.

Improper shoe cleat position or float increases the forces on your kneecaps as you pedal.

And if you don't have a helmet, get one.

Riding in gears that are too high or excessive hill climbing increases stress and exacerbates medial knee conditions. Anatomic abnormalities, such as genu varus, overpronation, internal tibial rotation, and hamstring tightness, may also exacerbate medial knee pain. Cyclists also need to be careful if they have problems with neck strain or other repetitive strain injuries of the upper extremities.

Stationary bikes are a great variation and one of my favorite workouts. I get to read or catch up on the news and break a great sweat. Bikes like Lifecycles offer a variety of workout options including interval training and hills. The stationary bike is also a cornerstone of knee rehabilitation because it is specific for building strength and endurance in the quadriceps muscle, so important for optimal knee health and function. But if you have patellar pain or significant weakness about your knee, start on "manual" for a flat ride, rather than attempting the hill profiles. Learn to use the pedal straps or toe clips, which make you more efficient and significantly reduce the forces across the knee.

GETTING WET

Water is an environment that's very forgiving for your frame, and even if you don't swim, there are water aerobics classes, as well as water yoga, Pilates, and Tai Chi for a low-impact workout. Buoyancy means that joint stresses are significantly lowered. When you're standing up to your neck in water, you weigh only 10 percent of what you do on land. Up to your chest, it's 25 percent; up to your waist, it's 50 percent. Variation in depth allows for a progression in stress levels for hopping and jumping drills for rehabilitation. Regaining lost joint motion and reducing swelling also seem to happen magically in a water environment.

At the Philadelphia 76ers' training facility, we have a submersible tank where the players can run, even on a stress fracture, while the AquaJogger and WetVest keep them buoyant. Kickboards and noodles are great, and you can use foot attachments and webbed gloves to make your routines harder and add "drag" resistance for strength building under water. There are even underwater bicycles.

Of course, the most common water workout—swimming—is not without its orthopaedic issues. Most high-level swimmers have been forced out of the water with rotator cuff problems at some point in their careers.

If you swim, do preventive work for your rotator cuff and also your neck, which is prone to problems or irritation. Also, know when to take a break.

Remember, too, that swimming doesn't count as strength training in terms of building your bones to prevent osteoporosis. The same buoyancy that makes water so forgiving means that you're getting a bit of a free ride like an astronaut in space. Without the pressure of gravity, your bones don't get the necessary stimulus to maintain themselves, so you'll still need to towel off and spend some time in the weight room.

AEROBICS CLASSES (HIGH AND LOW IMPACT)

In sports medicine, some of our steadiest repeat customers are aerobic dancers and their instructors, and this is even after the conversion to "low impact." Going from "high impact" classes to "low impact" simply means that shoulder strains and patellar pain have replaced foot and ankle injuries.

Lower impact doesn't always mean lower force. You fool yourself into thinking that it is a low-impact class, but if you are doing repetitive lunges, that's a "low-impact" that still creates tremendous cumulative forces across your patella. Skydiving, after all, is 99.9 percent floating on air, but I don't think anyone would call it low risk or low impact. That 0.1 percent can make a big difference, especially if you don't allow for adequate rest, recovery, or adaptation between sessions. Many aerobic studios have great carpet, but it's over concrete, which is just as bad as being on concrete itself. The ideal is a spring-floor, like a dance studio or a good basketball court. Even at the Pennsylvania Ballet, we worked out for a long time at two theaters with two different stages—one with more spring to it and one on a slant—and the dancers' injury patterns changed depending on which one they were using.

Often, when you ask somebody who does aerobic dance to cross-train, they want to run. But both activities create forces about the foot and ankle, and those stresses add up. Running and aerobics are not different activities in terms of giving your legs a rest.

True cross-training means that you run on some days, bike on other days, and perhaps swim on others. Tri-athletes are probably more heavily trained than a lot of the other single-sport athletes, but they have lower, not higher, injury rates. They spend less time in the repair shop because they mix things up, and the variety creates balance that is not present in predominately single-activity programs.

ALTERNATIVES FOR MAXIMIZING YOUR WORKOUT

In addition to the activities mentioned above, there are almost unlimited aerobic options.

Certainly martial arts and ballet are two of the greatest workouts. I would even put ice-skating on the list, along with skipping rope and shadow boxing. If you have a bad lower back, however, I would not recommend a rowing machine. If you have a bad neck and a bad shoulder, swimming makes less sense.

The elliptical cross-training machine is a great way to exercise your heart, especially if it ensures that you put in your 30 minutes, three times a week. Like stationary bicycles, the great advantage is that you can read. Let's face it; part of the challenge of tallying those aerobic minutes is boredom and time constraints. Try to find some things you like and some your frame tolerates, then mix and match.

INTERVAL TRAINING

Anything that makes your heart work harder, temporarily, will add to your level of aerobic conditioning, including increasing your pace or adding resistance. If you walk, throw in some jogging for 30 to 60 seconds. If you jog, add some sprint work. Increase the tension or level on your stationary bike or the step height on your stairclimber. Add some hills to your runs. "Intervals" can be incorporated into virtually any aerobic-type workout and will not only get you more fit, but they will also burn more calories and help prevent boredom. Incorporate intervals only after you are comfortable with your aerobic workout and even then, do it gradually

AEROBIC BOTTOM LINE

For optimal health and fitness, you need 30 minutes of aerobic or cardiovascular exercise at least three times a week. This can be done at the beginning of your FrameWork workout. Choose an aerobic activity for 30 minutes, which may include: cycling for 15 minutes, elliptical trainer for 15 minutes, or other options that add up to 30 minutes. Mix it up. If you already get your cardiovascular workouts elsewhere (for instance, you're a runner, swimmer, or tri-athlete), do a 12 to 15 minute aerobic activity (until you break a good sweat) to prepare your body for the work that follows.

THE MUSCLE IN THE MIDDLE (CORE STRENGTH AND FLEXIBILITY)

BALLET DANCERS, BOXERS, expert golfers, baseball sluggers, and practitioners of martial arts have long known that real power comes from the core of the body—the torso.

A strong core is the foundation for a balanced and optimal use of all musculature, lessening the chance of injury that comes when you strain to get power from just your arms or legs. Strengthening the core also dramatically lessens back problems. That's why this Step 3 of my FrameWork Program is all about strengthening your core.

The bible of core work are the writings of Joseph Pilates. But much of what we call "Pilates" today I learned from dancers in the early 1980s. I've used the techniques for more than 20 years in patient care.

The core is made up of several muscle groups, including the abdominal region (front-upper and lower and obliques), the lower back or spinal extensors, and muscles within the pelvic area. Especially important is the deeper abdominal muscle, the transverse abdominus, that attaches in the deeper areas near the spine. So working only those six-pack abs (the rectus abdominus front and center) will not build your core. In fact, if that's all you work, you'll be creating imbalances. You may look good in a Speedo, but your frame will be an accident waiting to happen.

If you think about it, your abdominal wall is the front of your back. The back extensors are the "back" of the back, and the oblique muscles come around the side. Strong abs protect the back, but doing abdominal exercises the wrong way (traditional situps, for instance) can do a lot more harm than good.

We now know that in terms of preventing back problems and back pain, the lumbar extensor muscles are probably the most important muscle group, but they are very hard to isolate and work. Most exercises meant to strengthen your back actually bring in other muscles, such as your gluteal (buttock) and upper hamstrings, which blunts the effectiveness of what you're trying to accomplish. If you aren't mindful about what you're doing, you can put a lot of time in, thinking you're working the lumbar extensors when actually you're not.

Arthur Jones, the original inventor of Nautilus and developer of the MedX line of equipment, kept trying to solve the problem of how to isolate the lumbar muscles and not have people leaning, or using their buttocks or their hamstrings to do that same movement. Your "cheatin' bod" always finds a way to make up for a weak link and fool you into thinking you are actually doing yourself good when in fact you are not. With the lower back, it happens all the time. MedX lumbar rehabilitation has helped many of my patients suffering with low back pain who have failed virtually every other treatment option.

Isolating and testing these muscle groups shows that the majority of people who suffer with chronic low back pain have problems with strength and endurance in their lower back extensor muscles. If you can deal with that and regain some of the strength and endurance in those muscles, you will resolve back pain in a majority of cases.

Once you strengthen them, lumbar extensors don't require the same amount of work as other muscle groups to maintain strength. You can get the job done working them once a week, or even once every two weeks.

Using the Swiss Ball or Thera-Ball, a firm, lightweight ball about the height of a chair—inexpensive and readily available—allows us to build core strength and balance by moderately engaging all the key torso musculature—abs, obliques, and back. When sitting "on the ball," your knees should be at approximately 90 degrees or just below the level of your hips. The balls come in different sizes for people of different heights:

5' to 5' 6"	55 cm
5' 7" to 6' 2"	65 cm
6' 3" and over	75 cm

As you go through this routine, focus intently on proper form. Our purpose is to help you derive the maximum benefit and to do the least harm. Even when the exercise seems familiar, doing it right actually makes it a very different experience. Also, when you see "OrthoCheck," I have provided pointers related to that particular exercise from an orthopaedic and rehabilitation standpoint to try to keep you out of trouble in terms of your frame and its vulnerabilities.

■ ■ ■ GETTING STARTED

Before jumping into the core exercises that follow, I recommend a cardiovascular (aerobic type) routine. If you perform regular cardiovascular exercise (you run, bike, swim, or walk), all you need is a 12 to 15 minute routine for a warm-up. You should at least break a sweat. If the FrameWork Program is your main cardiovascular exercise, then build up to 30 minutes of aerobic exercise. Either way, you should be fully warmed up before starting steps 3 (core) and 4 (powerful, pliable limbs).

Core exercises should be done with every workout. They should immediately follow your cardiovascular workout or warm-up. There are two core sequences you may choose from: one involves a mat routine (On the Mat) and the other a Swiss ball (On the Ball). Once you become comfortable with one, try substituting the other. Each core workout provides its own unique advantage.

ON THE MAT	ON THE BALL
Neck Roll	Neck Roll
Pillar Stretch	Pillar Stretch
Stork	Stork
Horse	Horse
Pelvic Tilt/Ab-Hollow	Spinal Extension (Passive Stretch)
Knee-to-Chest	Ball Crunch
Pretzel	Seated Twist
T-Roll	Seated Leg Extension
Crunch	Spinal Stretch (Thoracic Sag)
Cobra	Spinal Extension (Active)
Cat	
Child's Pose	
Superman	

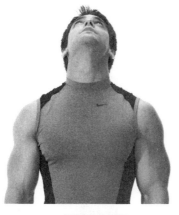

EXTENSION

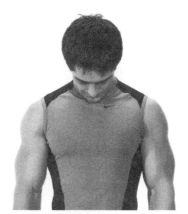

FLEXION

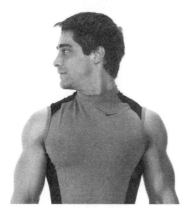

ROTATION

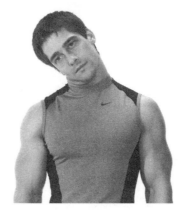

LATERAL BEND

Neck Roll

To improve neck range of motion

This is a variation of the original "neck roll," which is thought to place undo strain on the neck. This variation includes gaining neck mobility in three planes: flexion/extension, rotation, and lateral bending. Standing with your arms at your sides, look up, then down, then look to your right, tilt your head to your right. Then look to your left, tilt your head to your left.

Hold each for 5 seconds.

ORTHOCHECK

■ Gently and slowly perform the maneuvers.

■ Relax, breathe deeply.

■ Do not force or go beyond what is comfortable for you.

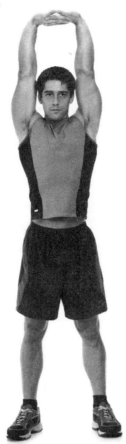

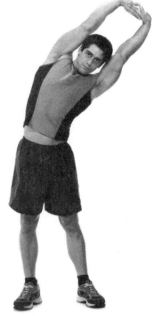

ADVANCED

Pillar Stretch

To improve shoulder mobility and rotator cuff function

Interlace fingers in front of you then turn palms outward and reach
straight for the sky, palms up until your hands are directly over your head
with your elbows straight.

Hold for 5 seconds.

■ **Advanced modification:** Alternate leaning gently to your left and
right during the hold.

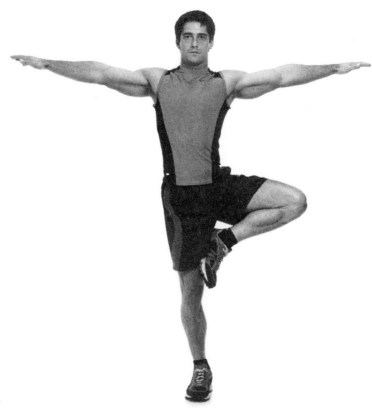

The Stork

To improve balance and body awareness

Stand up straight, extend your arms out wide to your sides, then raise one foot off the ground, up to the level of the opposite knee. Rest the arch of your foot on the inner side of your knee, forming the letter "P." Try not to sway or rock to maintain balance.

Hold for 10 seconds on each foot; try to build up to 20 seconds.

■ **Advanced modification:** As this gets easier, try to perform it with your eyes closed, on the ball of your foot, or on a small firm pillow.

This is a simple way to improve balance and will help with injury and fall prevention as well as improving sports performance. If you have had an injury (especially knee, foot, or ankle), this may be difficult, but it is an important part of your total recovery. If you have difficulty with this exercise, you should perform it several times per day, every day.

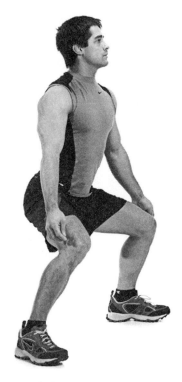

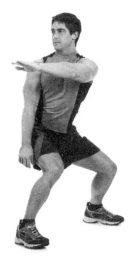

SIDE REACH MODIFICATION

The Horse

To improve leg (quad) strength and endurance

Start with your feet wider than shoulder-width apart, feet pointing forward. Staying tall, keeping your back and head straight and abdominal area tightened, begin to sink into a partial sitting position. Look straight ahead. Keep your knees outward, beyond your feet so that if you look down, your feet pointing straight ahead are on the inner side of your knees.

Hold for 20 seconds. Try to build up to a 1-minute hold.

■ **Modification:** As you improve the length of time holding this position, you can add the side-reach modification in which you twist your torso area and reach as far as possible to the left side with your right arm and alternate sides.

OrthoCheck

■ If you are unable to do the Horse because of pain or weakness, substitute a Wall Seat (on the opposite page). Hold for 20 seconds.

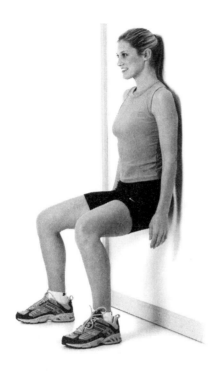

Wall Seat

To improve leg (quad) strength and endurance

Holding the Horse longer (5 to 10 minutes) is a great exercise and can be done several times per day.

If you have patellar pain syndrome with kneecap pain, then do a modified Horse or Wall Seat in a partial-sitting, partial-knee flexion position as your body allows. If you are unable to do these at all, you will need to work on quad isometrics daily until able to do a modified Horse or Wall Seat (for more information, see Patellar Pain Syndrome on page 217).

You should feel a burning sensation in the thigh muscle area (this is good) and not burning or pain in the kneecap area (not good).

ORTHOCHECK

■ It is great to combine it with a pelvic tilt or ab-hollow and relaxation breathing. Modification for patellar pain: Do not step out as far and only flex knee partially, that is, $\frac{1}{4}$ down. As you get stronger, you should gradually be able to go deeper. If you feel pain under the kneecap, you are going too deep. Sometimes there is a midrange of discomfort, and you actually can go deeper, beyond that of a comfortable position.

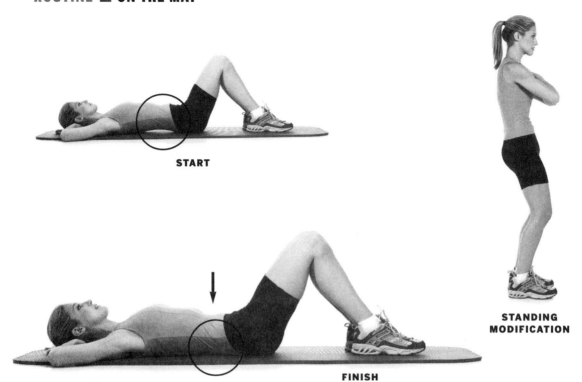

START

FINISH

STANDING
MODIFICATION

Pelvic Tilt/Ab-Hollow

For lower back health and core strength (Getting comfortable with this movement is important in preparing your body for much of the core training to follow.)

Lie on your back with your knees bent and feet flat on the floor. Pull in your stomach, bringing your belly button back toward your spine, tightening your abdominal area. Also gently tighten your gluteal/buttock muscles. Hold your abdominal area tight, concentrating on a spot approximately 2 inches deep to your belly button. You should feel the small of your back flatten toward the floor reversing the normal curve or arch in your lower back.

Hold this position for 6 to 10 seconds, then relax.
Repeat five times.

ORTHOCHECK:

■ If you have lower back problems, do this (either lying or standing version) often during the day. It can even be done sitting at your desk.

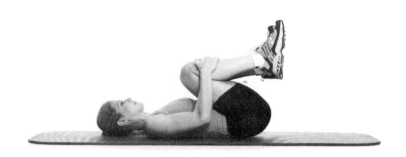

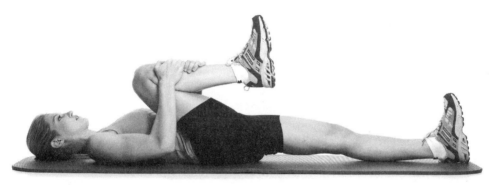

Knee-to-Chest

For lower back health and to improve hip mobility
Start with pelvic tilt and hold.

Pull your right leg/knee toward your chest with hands behind the knee area (or in front if it is more comfortable). Breathe comfortably during the stretch with relaxation breathing.

Relax, keeping your head on the floor.

Hold for 10 to 20 seconds. Repeat with left leg.

Next pull both knees to chest. Hold for 10 to 20 seconds.

OrthoCheck

■ **If you have neck problems, use a small pillow under your head.**

■ **If you have hip stiffness, bring your knees up only as far as is comfortable and try to improve this each time you perform the exercise.**

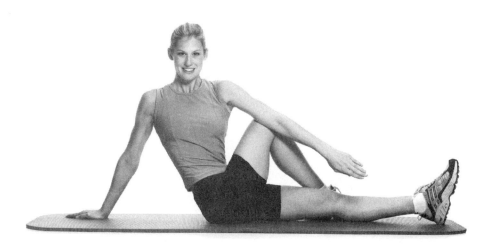

Pretzel

To improve lower back and trunk rotation, as well as outer hip and thigh flexibility

Sit with your left leg straight out and your right foot crossed over and just to the outside of your left knee. Place the outer side of your left elbow on the outer side of your right knee and thigh. Use your left elbow to pull your right knee inward (to the left) and lock it there. You should feel a stretch on the right outer hip and thigh area. Next, rotate your body around so you are looking over your right shoulder and even further behind you. This stretch is improved if you simultaneously lean into your knee with your left elbow and walk your right hand behind you on the floor as you bring yourself around. If you sit in the center of a room, with your back to the wall, you should try to look over your right shoulder to actually see the left corner behind you.

Hold for 10 to 20 seconds. Exhale as you slowly try to gain more movement. Repeat on opposite side.

■ A key is to feel a stretch in the upper outer thigh and hip area, and this is best accomplished by using your elbow to lever inward toward your knee while rotating far around to look as far behind you as possible, using the straightened arm behind you to assist with rotation.

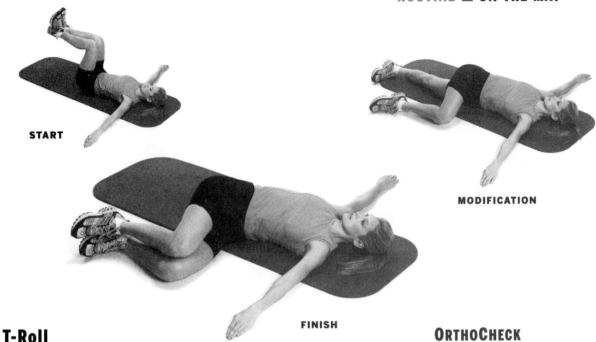

START

MODIFICATION

FINISH

T-Roll

Good for lower back and core-related flexibility

Lie on your back with legs straight and arms stretched out so that you form a "T." Bring both of your knees up so that your hips and knees are flexed to 90 degrees. Keeping the palms of your hands, elbows, and shoulders on the ground (don't let them lift off), twist your torso and rotate your pelvis and knees so that your left knee is on the ground by your side (keeping your knees together).

Hold for 5 to 7 seconds. Repeat on opposite side.

■ An alternate would be to do one leg at a time. Bring up one knee only, leaving the other leg straight out (or slightly) bent; use your opposite arm to help bring the knee toward the ground.

OrthoCheck

■ If your lower back and hips are tight, you many only be able to partially rotate and not have your knee reach the ground. Gradually try to improve how far you go.

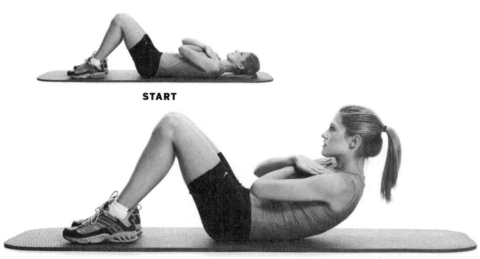

START

FINISH

Crunch

For abdominal and core strength as well as lower back health
Start with a pelvic tilt, tightening abs, knees bent, feet resting on floor.

Do not throw yourself forward.

Do not clasp your hands behind your head, but keep them near your ears, across your chest, or at your sides (with fingers pointing toward the knees, slide slowly forward and back approximately 4 to 6 inches as you go up and down).

Do not anchor your feet under anything or have someone hold your feet. This allows you to use your hip flexor muscles rather than your abs.

Tighten your abdominal muscle and slowly curl your head and shoulders off the floor; feel your breast bone accordian in toward your upper pubic bone. Pause momentarily and very slowly, in a controlled manner, come back down.

Do 10 repetitions.

ORTHOCHECK

■ **Don't bend your neck forward or tuck chin way into chest.**

■ **Don't come up past 30 degrees as you would in an old-fashioned situp.**

■ **You should feel the movement, the "burn" in your abs.**

■ **Keep your lower back pressed flat.**

■ **Concentrate on the feeling in your abs, and not how high you can lift off.**

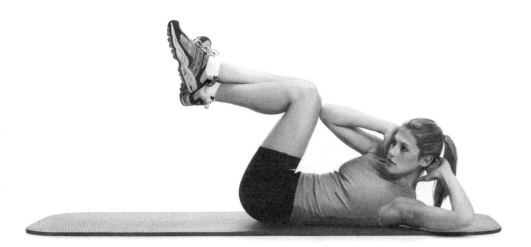

Crunch with Twist

Lie on your back with your ankles crossed and your hips and knees flexed at a 90-degree angle. Slowly perform a crunch, bringing your right elbow to your left knee.

Hold for 3 seconds. Do 10 repetitions and repeat on opposite side.

Use the same form as the basic crunch, i.e., pelvis tilt, slow movement up and down, and proper breathing. An easier alternative is to lie on your back with your right knee bent and foot resting on floor. Cross your left leg over your right knee. Keep left arm out on floor. Place your right hand near your right ear and slowly twist up bringing your right elbow toward your left knee.

■ In most gyms, there are great machine options for total abdominal work, and they include the ab machines or machine crunch as well as the rotary torso for obliques.

There are numerous alternatives that are worth incorporating in your workouts at various times. The basic crunch tends to work the upper abdominal area. To target your lower abdominal area, do a hanging knee raise from a chinup bar or do a reverse crunch. This can be done with your knees bent or straight for a more advanced option and your knees or legs are brought upward toward you. To target the obliques, you can perform a crunch with a twist, or try "Twist-Os (see page 233).

OrthoCheck

■ Slowly exhale during the lifting phase and inhale during the phase when you're lowering back to the floor.

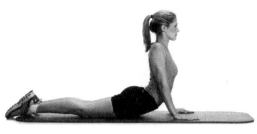

ADVANCED

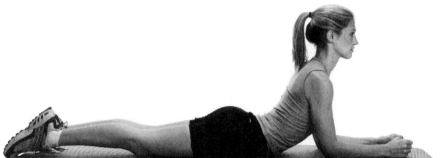

Cobra

For lower back flexibility (For those with bulging and herniated discs, this movement actually encourages your discs to move "back in place.")

Lie on your stomach. Slowly extend your back by propping up onto your elbows. Always keep the front of your hips and pelvis on the floor, don't let them lift off. Keep your neck in a comfortable position, especially if you have neck problems; don't look up.

Hold for 10 seconds; build up to 20 seconds.

■ **Advanced:** Once this is comfortable, progress to full Cobra position with arms almost fully extended (just shy of lockout position).

ORTHOCHECK

■ This exercise is very good for individuals with lower back disk problems (disk degeneration and disk herniation). If your facet joints, the smaller joints to either side of your disk area, are the problem, start by lying with your chest on a pillow, with your back in a slight extension. Gradually build up to resting on your elbows, progressing to the full cobra.

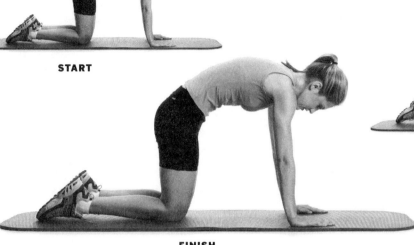

START

FINISH

MODIFICATION

Cat

For spinal mobility, especially thoracic and lumbar spine area
Kneel on the floor and support your weight on your palms in front of you, keeping your arms straight. Your knees should be just under your hips. Looking down, keep your neck relaxed and inhale, slowly pulling in your stomach. At the same time, arch your back upward as if a string is attached to your midback area, pulling it upward like a cat.
Hold for 5 seconds and repeat twice.

OrthoCheck

■ If you have lower back problems, you may not be able to lift as high, so work within your comfort range. Also, to help your lower back, after you return to the starting position, try the knee to chest alternate: Tighten your abdominal area, gently lift one knee toward your chest, hold for several seconds; repeat with the opposite side. This gently stretches your lower back and thoracic area.

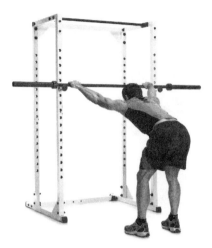

STANDING MODIFICATION

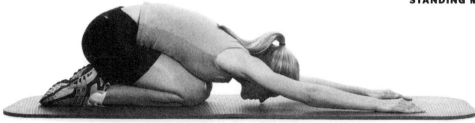

Child's Pose

For spine and shoulder mobility

After completing the cat, rise back to a kneeling position. Gently sit back onto your heels (or as far as you can comfortably go). Lower your forehead and chest area toward the floor as your arms (palms down) reach forward. Slide your palms forward as far as they will go, feeling both a relaxation and stretch in the spine, latissimus, and shoulder area. **Hold for 5 seconds.**

■ **Standing modification:** Lean forward along a Smith machine or countertop with your arms straight out while bending at the waist and looking downward. Gently rock your hips and pelvis backward so that you feel a stretch in the upper back, lat, and shoulder area.

ORTHOCHECK

■ If your knees won't bend far enough, try this with a pillow under your buttocks.

■ If your lower back is tight or uncomfortable, start with your knees wider apart. If because of lower back, hip, or knee problems Child's Pose is not yet possible, try the standing modification.

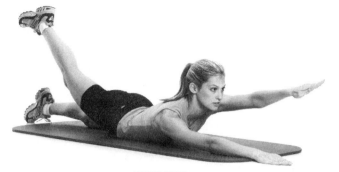

BEGINNER

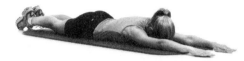

MODIFIED START

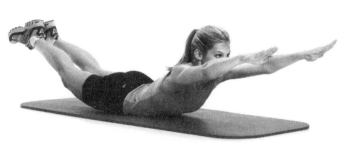

ADVANCED

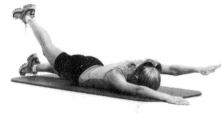

MODIFICATION

Superman

For spinal extensor muscle strength and overall spine health
Start lying on the floor facedown with your arms straight out. (Picture
Superman flying in the air.)

Raise left arm and right leg off ground. Keep your knees straight so that
your legs are being lifted by buttocks and lower back. If it does not bother
your neck, your head should also come off the ground.
Hold 10 seconds and build up to 20 seconds. Alternate sides.

■ **Advanced:** Simultaneously bring both of your arms and both legs off
of the ground. Only your abdominal area and pelvis should be on the
ground.
Hold for 10 seconds and build up to 20 seconds. Repeat 3 times.

OrthoCheck

■ If you have neck
problems, you can
keep your face
resting on the ground
and not lift your
head.

■ If you are unable
to do even the
beginner version, you
can start with just
lifting any one arm or
leg off the ground
and build up to the
beginner and then
more advanced
versions.

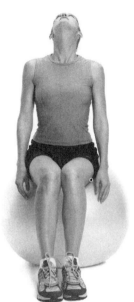

EXTENSION

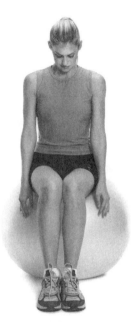

FLEXION

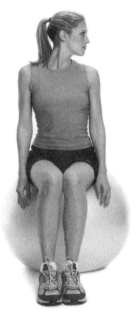

ROTATION

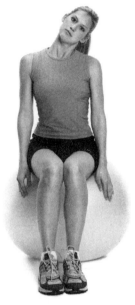

LATERAL BEND

Neck Roll

To improve neck range of motion

This is a variation of the original "neck roll," which is thought to place undo strain on the neck. This variation includes gaining neck mobility in three planes: extension/flexion, rotation, and lateral bending.

Standing with your arms at your sides, look up, then down, then look to your right, tilt your head to your right. Then look to your left, tilt your head to your left.

Hold each for 5 seconds.

ORTHOCHECK

■ Gently and slowly perform the maneuvers.

■ Relax, breathe deeply.

■ Do not force or go beyond what is comfortable for you.

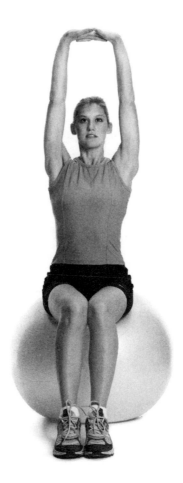

Pillar Stretch

To improve shoulder mobility and rotator cuff function

Interlace your fingers in front of you then turn your palms outward and reach straight for the sky, palms up until your hands are directly over your head with your elbows straight.

Hold for 5 seconds.

■ Alternate leaning gently to your right and left during the hold.

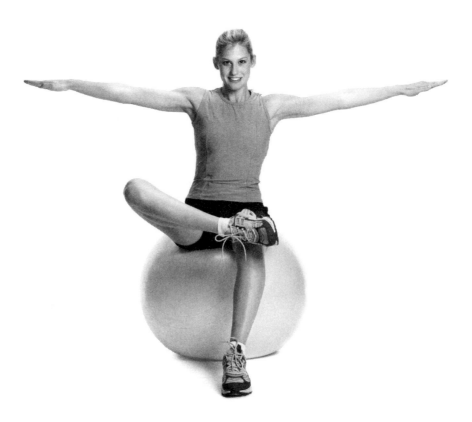

The Stork

To improve balance and body awareness

Sit on ball. Cross right leg over left knee. Extend arms out to sides.
Try not to sway or rock to maintain balance.

Hold for 10 seconds on each foot. Try to build up to 20 seconds.

■ **Advanced:** As this gets easier, try to perform it with your eyes closed,
on the ball of your foot.

This is a simple way to improve balance and will help with injury and fall
prevention as well as improving sports performance.

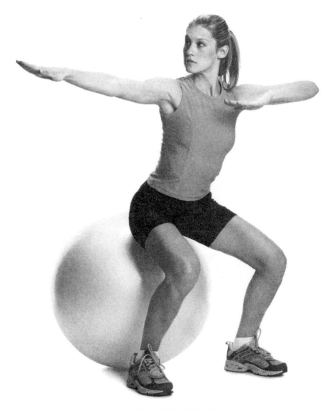

SIDE REACH VERSION

The Horse

To improve leg (quad) strength and endurance

Start with your feet wider than shoulder-width apart, feet pointing forward. Staying tall, keeping your back and head straight and abdominal area tightened, begin to sink into a partial sitting position so you are barely sitting on the ball. Look straight ahead. As you advance, you may add the neck and body rotation (as shown above). Keep your your knees outward, beyond your feet so that if you look down, your feet pointing straight ahead are on the inner side of your knees. As you improve the length of time holding this position, you can add the side-reach modification in which you twist your torso area and reach as far as possible to the right and alternate sides.

Hold for 20 seconds.

ORTHOCHECK

■ If you are unable to do the Horse because of pain or weakness, substitute a Wall Seat (see page 79) or try sitting partially on the ball until you build up enough strength.

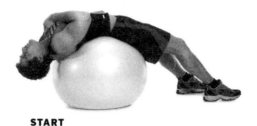

START

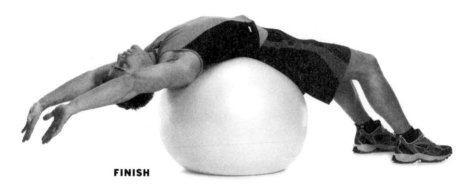

FINISH

Spinal Extension (Passive Stretch)

Stretches and relaxes entire spine and is excellent for posture, especially for people who tend to hunch forward or who have a thoracic kyphosis in which the mid to upper spine is flexed forward Start by sitting on the ball, with your feet on the floor. Slowly step forward, letting the ball roll backward to your lower back area so that your back arches backward over the ball. Lie back, initially keeping your arms crossed on chest. Next try reaching backward, opening up your shoulders, reaching toward the floor behind you.

Hold for 10 seconds.

■ You can slightly roll back and forth to improve the stretch and massage the spinal area.

■ **Advanced:** As you improve your spinal mobility, you can advance to where your hands reach back to touch the floor.

ORTHOCHECK

■ If help is needed getting up, bring your arms forward to the chest area.

■ If you have neck problems or symptoms, use your hands behind your neck area to gently help lift up and support the neck area during this exercise.

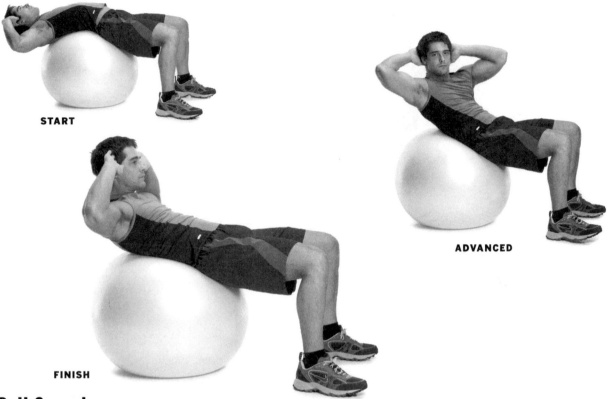

START

FINISH

ADVANCED

Ball Crunch

For abdominal and core strength

Lie on the ball with your hands near your ears or across your chest, feet resting on the floor. Tighten and hollow your abs, slowly curl up, concentrating on using your abs so that your head and shoulders come up to a position that is approximately halfway between lying and sitting. **Hold for 5 seconds. Roll back slowly to the starting position, keeping your abs tight all the way back. Repeat 10 times.**

■ **More advanced:** Allow yourself to start from a position further back over the ball (i.e., step backward and let the ball roll forward slightly under you).

■ **More advanced alternative:** Ball crunch with twist.

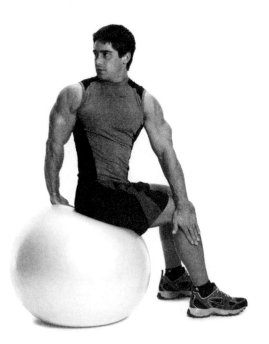

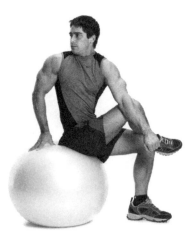

ADVANCED

Seated Twist

For spinal and torso mobility

Sit tall on the ball with your feet on the ground, tighten your abs, place your left hand on the outer side of of your right knee/thigh. Rotate at the spine, gently pushing at the spine and gently pushing with left hand to help turn your spine and shoulders so you are looking behind as you reach behind with your right arm (steady ball with left hand if needed to assist).

Hold for 5 seconds and alternate sides.

■ **More advanced alternative:** Same movement with legs crossed and resting on opposite knee area.

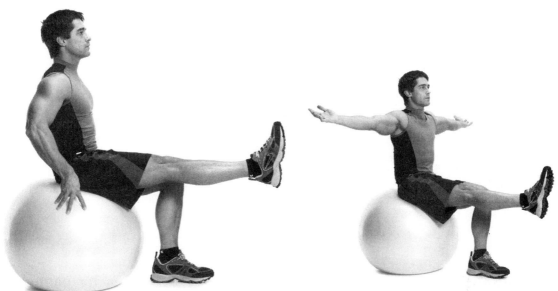

Seated Leg Extension

For balance, quadriceps and hamstring strength, and hamstring flexibility

Sit on the ball, tall and upright, with your feet no more than shoulder-width apart and your hands resting on the side of the ball. Tighten your abdominal muscles. Keeping your left foot flat on the floor, extend your right leg fully, tightening your thigh muscle.

Hold for 10 seconds and alternate sides. Repeat each side 5 times.

■ **More advanced:** Remove your hands from the ball and keep them out to the sides forming a "T."

■ For even more of a challenge, add ankle weights. Start with 1 or 2 pounds. Also, try doing this while on the ball of your foot, rather than keeping your foot flat on the floor.

ORTHOCHECK

■ If your hamstrings are tight, you will not be able to fully straighten your leg but go to where it is comfortable and hold that position, trying to improve each time.

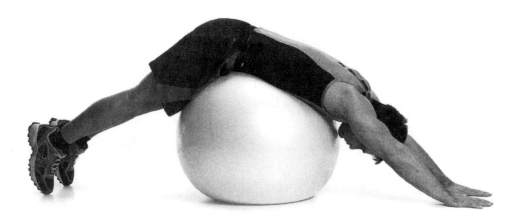

Spinal Stretch (Thoracic Sag)

To stretch entire spine (especially lower back) and buttock and hamstring area and also help reverse lumbar lordosis (tightness of lower back causing lower back to arch in many people).
Hold for 10 to 20 seconds.

ORTHOCHECK

■ If uncomfortable, start with Drape, which is a "tighter" version of this exercise with your hands and feet closer to the ball. You can even start kneeling on the ground, hugging the ball. Progress to where your knees are off the ground but remain slightly flexed and closer to the ball. As flexibility, stability, and balance improve, you can progress to the full Spinal Stretch.

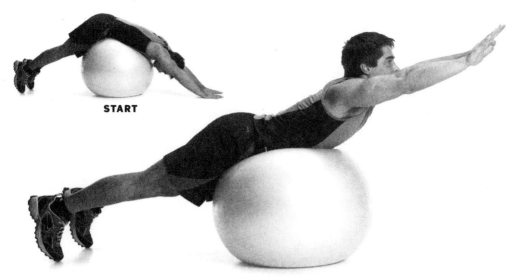

START

FINISH

Spinal Extension (Active), "Superman" on the ball

For spinal extensor muscle strength and endurance and gluteal (buttock) strength

From the Spinal Stretch position, keeping your feet on ground and legs straight, slowly extend your lumbar area until you are straight or slightly extended in the lower back area and your arms are fully extended outward like Superman flying.

Hold for 10 seconds and build up to 20 seconds.

■ **More advanced alternative:** Get into the Superman position and then gently lift one leg off the ground while fully straight, balancing only on the opposite straightened leg. This further strengthens the gluteal or buttock area. Hold 5 seconds then alternate legs.

■ **An even more advanced version:** While in the Superman position, use your feet to gently propel you forward so that you then land on your outstretched hands with your feet in the air. Push backward with your hands to get back to the starting position.

■ **Most advanced version:** Do the full Superman in which only your abdominal area is on the ball and both feet and arms are outward in the "flying" position.

ORTHOCHECK

■ If you are unable to perform this, start where you assist yourself by keeping your hands on the floor and just slightly lifting them off the floor when possible. Gradually build up to where you can straighten your back fully and then start bringing your hands upward to the full Superman.

MUSCLES ARE SHOCK ABSORBERS. After the age of forty, the average person loses muscle mass at the rate of 1 percent a year, but some do it even more rapidly, and some begin well before 30. Less shock absorption means more joint stresses and less joint protection, which means a less durable you.

Muscle also drives metabolism—it's a furnace for burning calories—so even if your food intake remains steady, less muscle can mean a midsection that expands far more quickly than your stock portfolio. The good news, of course, is that this muscle loss is preventable, similar to the bone loss attributed to osteoporosis.

The right kind of exercise prevents muscle loss by tipping the balance of catabolic (tearing down) and anabolic (building up) processes toward the latter. Muscle that is worked to exhaustion, then properly nourished and allowed to rest, rebuilds itself larger and stronger than it was before.

But our objective isn't just to be big and strong. We want to be built to last. That's why we fully integrate strength training *and* flexibility training within the same program. Otherwise, time constraints usually means scrimping on one or the other, and one without the other is an engraved invitation to injury.

Strengthening and stretching are too important to be done in a "hit-and-run" fashion. It takes concentration to really work the entire muscle. And to "first, do no harm" requires that you *control* the forces you apply.

Physics tells us that force is related to mass (amount of weight) multiplied by velocity *squared*. In plain English—by increasing the velocity or speed of movement, you increase the risk of creating damaging forces. The damage can occur both suddenly (obvious muscle or tendon tear), or it can be more subtle, with gradual wear and tear (silent but very common) taking its toll over time, resulting in a weakened, vulnerable frame. To avoid injury, you have to take your time—avoiding bouncy movements and raising and lowering the weights s-l-o-w-l-y.

Even if jerky movements don't send you immediately to the ice pack (or the ER), they will contribute to strength curve imbalances. Remember the NHL goalie? Jerking the weight up and down also deprives you of the eccentric or negative part of the lift, an essential stimulus for optimal muscle growth and strengthening.

If you're trying to improve your performance in a sport by developing sudden bursts of strength, that's a project for the playing field, not the weight room. Moving weights faster won't make you faster, but it may sideline you indefinitely.

As for the amount of weight, my general observation is that most men should probably try using less, and most women should probably try using more. The men who use too much are trying to demonstrate strength rather than build it; the women who use too little are often afraid of turning into the Incredible Hulk. But as we've said before, there's really no physiological reason for women to fear that they'll get bulky. Barring some major hormonal imbalance, it just isn't going to happen.

Twelve to 15 reps is usually the right number to completely exhaust the muscle—which is the objective. If you can get to 15 reps consistently, then it's time to progress to slightly heavier loads, either by adding more weight, or by increasing the resistance of your elastic tubing.

But before increasing your weight, do a few workouts where you slow the lift/lower movement even more to really stimulate the muscle and recruit muscle fibers for optimal growth. Going very s-l-o-w increases the challenge, which increases the benefit.

You want to work each muscle to "failure," meaning that you cannot complete the repetition. But one thing you have to watch out for is shoulder pain—very common in the weight room—related to a combination of positional overload, muscle imbalance, and the "weak link" phenomenon. You can have huge, strong deltoid muscles draping the shoulders, as big as football pads, and still have weakness—even difficulty lifting the arm overhead—if the tiny rotator cuff strap muscle group in your shoulder is malfunctioning. Exercises to strengthen the shoulder/deltoid will only increase the problem. That's why we offer very specific shoulder stretching, combined with rotator cuff strengthening and modified shoulder limited arc lifts, all aimed at repair, recovery, and—better yet—prevention.

RELEASING YOUR INNER GUMBY (STRETCHING)

When I was in training at the University of Pennsylvania, the Penn Relays, held every spring, drew track and field athletes from all over the world. On beautiful days, you'd see the runners out there early, taking warmup laps and lying down on the ground to stretch. In Philadelphia in the spring, however, we get a lot of rain. And on rainy days, in every race, you'd see a runner break stride and be left behind, grabbing his leg as if he'd been shot—the telltale sign of a hamstring pull. I don't think it had anything to do with running on a wet track. I think it's that on rainy days, the runners didn't take the time to warm up and get down on the ground to stretch their muscles.

For most people, stretching is the most neglected area of their exercise routines. We all need to stretch more, but keep in mind that warming up and stretching are two different activities, and you need to do both.

Muscle tightness is the indicator most closely linked to specific injury patterns. Tight quadriceps predisposes for jumper's knee. A tight calf leads to Achilles tendinitis and heel pain. Hamstring tightness can lead to low back pain and patellar problems. And among our weekend warriors in their forties and fifties, playing in winter basketball and summer softball leagues, one of the most common ailments I see is a pull or tear in the medial gastroc muscle (the bulge just below the knee on the back of the leg), which can happen to anyone with tight calves.

Not only is tightness an invitation to injury, but you'll never get peak performance with tight muscles restricting your movement.

But even people who recognize the importance of stretching too often think of it as a warmup. Stretching isn't a preliminary to be hurried out of the way; it's part of the main event. Equally important, you need to warm up *before* you stretch.

Walk around the track a few times, first, or jog lightly to get your blood flowing. Try to break a sweat, or at least get your face flushed. Give your collagen time to loosen up.

This workout integrates strengthening and stretching because, whenever you have a flexibility/strength mismatch, you're at risk for a muscle or joint injury. You need strong muscles around that joint to keep everything in place and to provide muscle control through the full range of movement.

Some people are inherently more flexible than others because their collagen is more elastic. But being naturally loose jointed can be too much of a good thing. There are people who have Ehlers-Danlos Syndrome, a collagen disease, which produces a range from super flexibility to "circus contortionist."

Women tend to be a little more loose jointed and flexible than guys, which means they need to spend more time in the gym, even if that means less time in yoga class. Guys who are muscular probably need to shift some of their time in the weight room toward time doing yoga or other stretching. People who run, swim, or bike for mile after mile need to break up their routines with some weight training and stretching. In the end, it's all about balance.

TOO MUCH OF A GOOD THING

A ballerina who can get her leg into an extreme position needs muscle control that serves her in that extended range of motion. Otherwise, she's prone to either sudden or cumulative trauma to her joints and supporting tissues, and even more so when fatigue or dehydration sets in. Likewise, gymnasts and ice skaters who can do those beautiful back bends, lowering their heads back until they almost reach their hips, have high incidences of stress fractures in their lower backs. Once you go back that far, your soft tissue allows you to go there, but the bone now is absorbing higher stresses than it can tolerate. Sometimes this leads to a condition called spondylolisthesis, in which one vertebrae starts to slip in relation to the other. The only protection is to have great core strength, so that the muscles are in control of the fine movements, with stability instead of bone-on-bone contact.

PROPRIOCEPTIVE NEUROMUSCULAR FACILITATION (PNF) STRETCHING

PNF is an aid to stretching that's especially effective for stubborn tight areas, "tight" individuals, or those with recurrent muscle pulls. Variations include:

The contract-relax technique

Normally, when you stretch a muscle, it reaches a limit; it just won't go any further without tearing or straining. But when you contract and tighten that same muscle prior to the stretch, the contraction acts like a circuit breaker, momentarily overriding your muscle-tightening capabilities. It also adjusts your stretch reflex involving stretch receptors in the muscle. When the muscle is relaxed after that contraction, it momentarily has a new "set point" of limitation and is able to safely elongate or lengthen more.

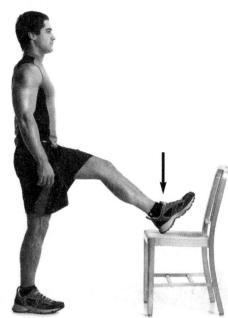

HAMSTRING PNF STRETCH

Take the hamstring as an example. Place your straight right leg on a chair or firm bench with the heel resting on the surface. Isometrically tighten your hamstring muscle by pulling down on your heel as if you were trying to press the top of the chair downward, keeping the leg straight or only slightly flexed. Hold this tightly for 10 seconds and feel the back of your thigh/hamstring to ensure it is tightening. Next, relax the muscle and immediately go into a hamstring stretch, holding for 10 to 15 seconds. To avoid raising your blood pressure, be sure to breathe comfortably throughout this exercise, especially with the isometric muscle hold.

The antagonist contract-relax technique

When you contract one muscle (i.e., quadriceps or biceps) your body automatically relaxes the opposing antagonist muscle (i.e., hamstrings or triceps).

Again, for the hamstring, first tighten your quadriceps muscle either by straightening your knee fully and tightening the front of the thigh or by bringing your knee forward and resisting that motion with your hands while pushing up on your knee area. This movement will facilitate your hamstring's relaxation by a "reciprocal inhibition reflex." As soon as you relax your front thigh muscle, you can immediately go into a stretch of the rear thigh or hamstring.

PNF techniques work especially well when used as a partner stretch, where someone assists you with the movement. Your partner, however, needs to be careful not to force any movements. Before many pro games begin, you can often see athletes lying on the field or court with their trainers going through some of these maneuvers. Chances are you won't need them for every muscle group, but most of us could use a

PNF technique for certain stubborn muscle groups. PNF techniques are especially useful around the shoulder, hips, and hamstring areas.

In the regime that follows, I've interspersed strengthening and stretching exercises, blending them to create a natural flow from one routine to the next. If done properly—without too much stopping to chat or check out who's looking good in their Spandex across the gym—the routine also keeps your heart rate elevated for an extended period of time, improving your aerobic conditioning while you're gaining both strength and flexibility.

Remember, not everyone is a Gumby, and stretching is not a competition. Your goal is not to be as loose-jointed as your yoga instructor or a prima ballerina, but rather to improve your flexibility a little each day. Stretching is also a very effective relaxation technique. For a more extensive approach to stretching techniques, a book I recommend to every athlete and active individual—especially those with tight muscles—is Bob Anderson's *Stretching,* a classic.

■ ■ ■ RANGE OF MOTION

Every joint in your body has a unique path of movement as you bend fully (flexion) and straighten fully (extension). This is called range of motion or ROM, and your body is usually right and left symmetrical in this regard. Variations in ROM, left to right, or serious loss of ROM, can be related to prior injuries or other joint conditions such as arthritis. Early ROM loss can be very subtle and not even noticeable, especially since your body makes adjustments and compensates, hiding the problem from you at first—until other problems show up elsewhere down the line.

■ ■ ■ GETTING STARTED

The FrameWork strengthening and stretching routine can be done anywhere. If you go to the gym I provide a machine (or cable) circuit. It can also be done with free weights or even elastic tubing. Choose one of the three columns below, depending on your circumstance.

For exercises that may not be familiar to you, I provide detailed explanations and for those that are well known, the photos will suffice. If you go to the gym and use machines, the trainers or instructors will be able to help you navigate the routine.

As with the core exercises (which should precede these), you should be warmed up and sweating before starting. Remember to lift weights slowly (4 count up—pause momentarily—4 count down) and never sacrifice form for amount lifted. Stretching should be slow and without bounce usually holding for 10 to 20 seconds.

GYM—MACHINES OR CABLE UPPER BODY	GYM/HOME—FREE WEIGHTS UPPER BODY	HOME—TUBING ETC. UPPER BODY
Lat Pulldown	One-Arm Dumbbell Row	Lat Pulldown
Climb the Rope	*Climb the Rope*	*Climb the Rope*
Machine Row	One-Arm Dumbbell Rear Cuff Row	Bow and Arrow
Arm Cross Stretch	*Arm Cross Stretch*	*Arm Cross Stretch*
Upright Row	Upright Row	Upright Row
Lateral Raise	Dumbbell Lateral Raise	Lateral Raise
Pec Machine	Bench Press	Push-ups
Doorjamb Stretch	*Doorjamb Stretch*	*Doorjamb Stretch*
Biceps Curl	Biceps Curl	Biceps Curl
Triceps Extension	One-Arm Triceps Kickback	Triceps Extension
TriSho Stretch	*TriSho Stretch*	*TriSho Stretch*
Forearm Strength	Forearm Strength	Forearm Strength
Forearm Stretch	*Forearm Stretch*	*Forearm Stretch*

LOWER BODY	LOWER BODY	LOWER BODY
Knee Extension	Leg Lift with Ankle Weight	Tubing Leg Extension
Quad Stretch	*Quad Stretch*	*Quad Stretch*
Leg Press	Squat	Tubing Squat
Leg Curls	One-Leg Curls with Ankle Weight	Tubing Kickback
Ham Stretch	*Ham Stretch*	*Ham Stretch*
Ab and Add Machine	One-Leg Ab and Add with Weight	Tubing Ab and Add
Straddle Stretch	*Straddle Stretch*	*Straddle Stretch*
Psoas Stretch	*Psoas Stretch*	*Psoas Stretch*
Calf Raise	Calf Raise	Calf Raise
Calf Stretch	*Calf Stretch*	*Calf Stretch*

NOTE: Stretches are italicized.

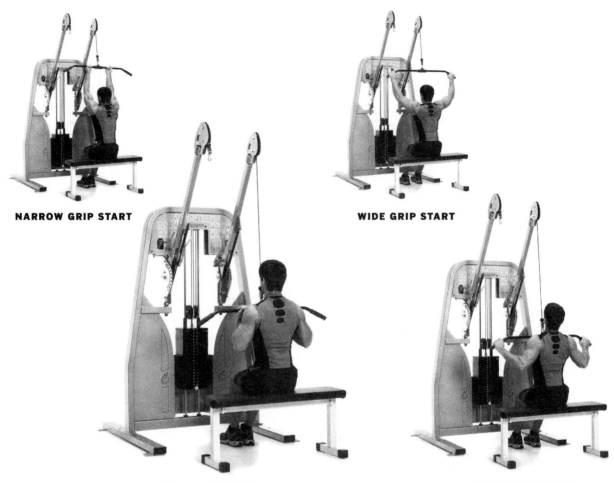

NARROW GRIP START

WIDE GRIP START

NARROW GRIP FINISH

WIDE GRIP FINISH

Lat Pulldown

Builds a strong upper back and "V"-shape; also helps prevent shoulder shoulder problems.

Can be done with a wide grip, palms out or a more narrow grip, palms in (my preference) or one arm at a time (with tubing or pulley).

As you pull down, there is a tendency to lean back. Slight leaning is okay but don't use the momentum of leaning back to assist the movement; it cheats the lats. Concentrate on using your lats to do the work. Slowly bring the bar to your breast bone area.

OrthoCheck

■ I don't like the behind-the-neck lat pulldown, which all too often irritates the neck and shoulder areas.

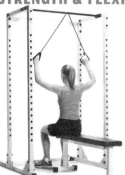

TUBING START

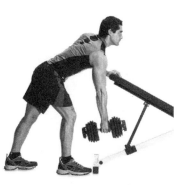

ONE-ARM DUMBBELL ROW START

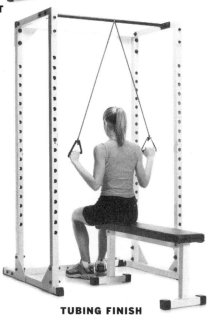

ONE-ARM DUMBBELL ROW FINISH

TUBING FINISH

■ **Alternate:** Freeweight version is the one-arm dumbbell row and the tubing version is a tubing lat pulldown.

■ **Alternate:** Chinups are a great alternative and can also be done as "negative" chinups.

■ **If you have shoulder impingement or rotator cuff issues, the wide grip with palms out sometimes pinches or irritates the shoulder.**

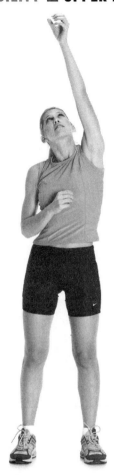

Climb the Rope

For shoulder, latissimus, and spinal mobility

While looking slightly up, tighten your abdominal area (suck it in doing an Ab-Hollow maneuver). Reach way up with your left hand, then reach even higher; cross your right hand over the left as if you were climbing a rope (really reaching is important). You should feel it in your shoulders and upper back. Done correctly, this is excellent for posture and works the entire spinal area and abdominal obliques for both strength and flexibility. Do three repetitions on each side.

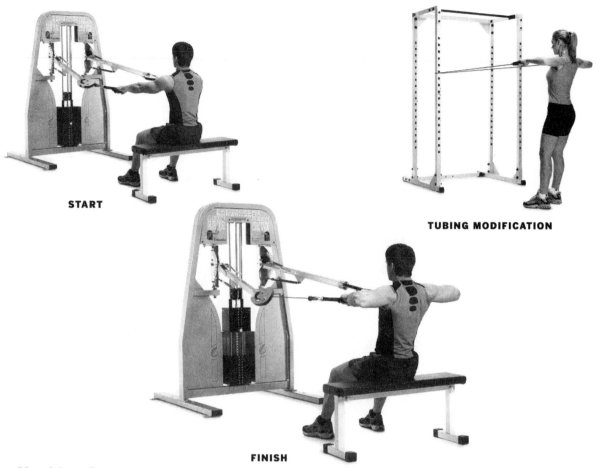

START

TUBING MODIFICATION

FINISH

Machine Row

Improves posture and important for rotator cuff health and function

If you are doing these properly, you don't need much weight. The body cheats by bringing in momentum (by moving too fast) and also by having your elbows drop slightly down, which brings in your lats rather than working the rear shoulder, rear cuff, and scapular (shoulder blade) stabilizer.

Keep your elbows high (at shoulder level throughout entire movement) and lead backward with the elbow tip, imagining a string attached to the elbow pulling it backward. You should feel the muscle working behind your shoulder and around your shoulder blade.

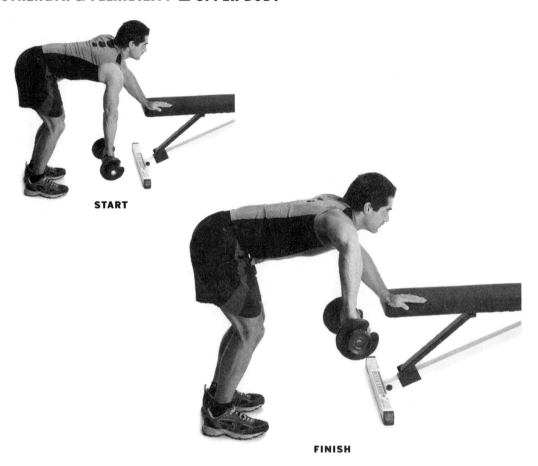

START

FINISH

One-Arm Dumbbell Rear Cuff Row

Lean on bench, keeping your back flat. Don't bob up and down. Your elbow and arm should be the only things moving. Keeping the elbow at the same level as the shoulder (not dropping downward), lead with your elbow upward. Imagine a string pulling the elbow toward the ceiling.

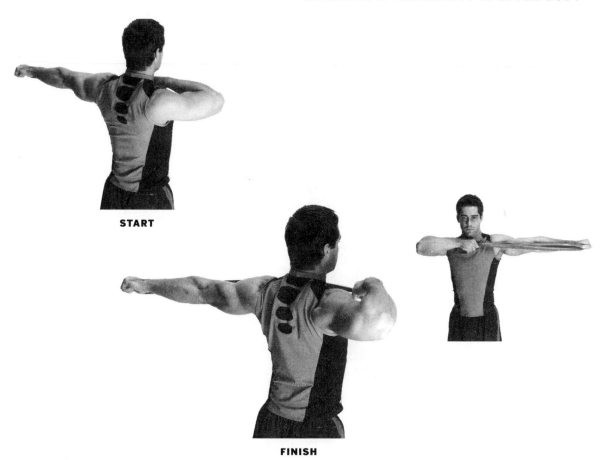

START

FINISH

Bow and Arrow

Start with elastic tubing held tightly with the left arm extended and the right hand in front of the chest. Keeping your right elbow higher than your right shoulder, pull back on the tubing with the right hand but actually feel the motion lead from the right elbow heading backward. Pull until you are in the fully extended position as if you were squeezing your shoulder blades together, also pulling both shoulders backward. Your left hand and right elbow should be slightly behind the plane of your shoulders, and you should feel a slight stretch in the chest area.

OrthoCheck

■ If you have shoulder difficulties, start extremely light with the tubing so this movement is easy. If there is discomfort in the shoulder, you may need to slightly drop your elbow as you pull back.

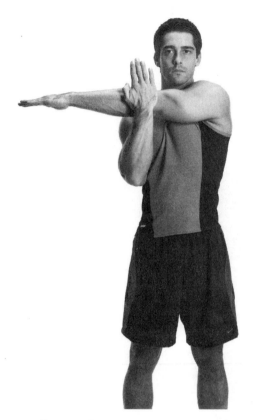

Arm Cross Stretch

Improves rear shoulder and rotator cuff flexibility

Fully straighten your left arm in front of you and place your right fist above the left elbow. Using your right arm, pull your left arm across your chest so your forearm is hitting toward your right shoulder. Go until you can't go any further (you should feel a stretch behind the left shoulder) and hold for 10 seconds. Don't let your elbow drop down, stay high, just below your chin. Then, keeping your arm in this stretched position, let your left elbow flex so you give yourself a hug or a pat on the back. As you improve, you should be able to reach farther across your back. Alternate sides.

■ **Hold for 10 seconds and then immediately go into the stretch position.**

OrthoCheck

■ If you have tight shoulders or rotator cuff problems, you may want to add a PNF version. Before you pat yourself on the back, try pushing back with your right elbow into your left fist but don't allow your arm to move. Then stretch.

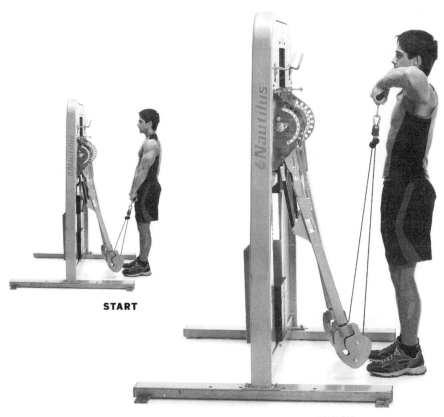

START

FINISH

Upright Row

Keep your neck relaxed, avoiding the tendency to tighten it backward, especially if you have neck problems. There is a tendency, especially if you're lifting too much weight, to tighten and compress the neck area.

■ **Alternate:** The free-weight version can be with a barbell or two dumbbells. The tubing version can be done while standing on the elastic tubing.

OrthoCheck

■ If you have shoulder problems, keep the weight lower and do the first three or four reps going only to the breast bone area; then with each rep come a little higher. Also try moving hands closer together.

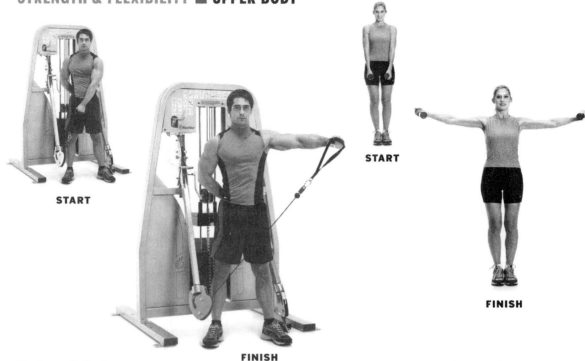

START

FINISH

START

FINISH

Lateral Raise

Keeping your elbows slightly bent, slowly raise your arm outward until arm is parallel to ground or slightly higher (don't force it too high). As you are lifting, slightly tilt the thumb side of your hand downward (as if you are pouring out just a little water from a bottle). This better isolates the mid and rear deltoid and rotator cuff (the front deltoid gets plenty of work with other upper body exercises, in fact it is often overworked). Pause momentarily and slowly let the weight down to the starting point. Don't tighten your neck, pulling it back during the lift, which causes neck strain.

■ **Modification:** Applies to all exercises (i.e., machines, tubings, free-weights). If you have shoulder or neck problems, do this one arm at a time while supporting yourself. This better isolates the working shoulder and removes any unnecessary neck strain or compression. It also makes cheating with momentum less likely. Also, with shoulder problems, do not lift as high. Go just below 90 degrees, keeping your hand below the level of your shoulder until this gets more comfortable, then gradually go higher as tolerated.

ORTHOCHECK

■ If shoulder problems make lateral raises too uncomfortable, shorten the arc so that you are only lifting off at about 45 degrees until your shoulders improve. If it is impossible to do even modified lateral raises, focus more time and effort on the rotator cuff rotation exercises and plan (page 210).

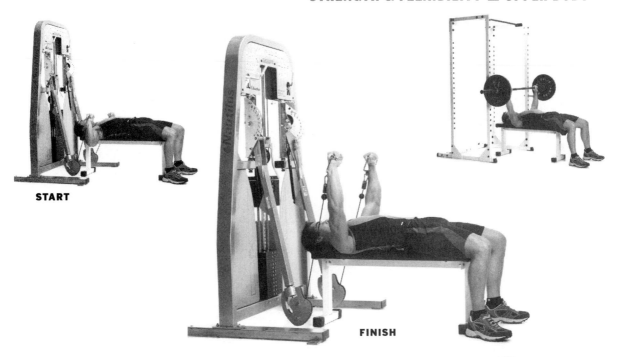

START

FINISH

Pec Machine Bench Press

Don't arch your back or lift your buttocks off the bench. Don't bounce the weights off your chest. It may feel good and allow you to use more weight, but it can be dangerous to your shoulders with either a sudden injury or, more commonly, low-grade cumulative damage over time. Don't lock out your elbows (especially suddenly). Be sure to tighten your abdominal area during the lift and don't hold your breath.

■ **Alternate:** Dips are a great alternative or addition and be sure to include "negative" dips. If you can do 15 dips without difficulty in good form, consider adding some weight. Certain machines have this capability with a strap around the waist, or you can add ankle weights.

■ **Modification:** If you have shoulder symptoms with the bench press, try different angles (i.e., incline or decline) or vary the grip on the barbell. A wider grip works more of the chest area and a more narrow grip works more of the triceps. Vary to see what is comfortable for you. Also, use a pec machine if available and "pin the stack" so your arm does not go back as far. This is especially important for those with shoulder instability who either sublux or dislocate their shoulders.

ORTHOCHECK

■ If you have low back problems, it helps to rest your feet on the bench with your knees flexed.

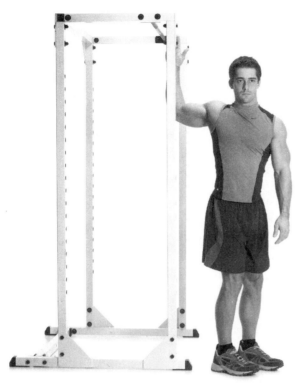

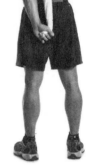

TOWEL STRETCH

Doorjamb Stretch

The front of the shoulder and pectoral area are extremely common areas of tightness in most individuals, and this stretch should be done regularly even on days when you are not at the gym.

The key is to keep your elbow at the same height as your shoulder, and when you lean inward, picture yourself leading first with the front of the shoulder arching inward. Keep your palm open and holding on the doorjamb.

■ **PNF modification:** This is a great area for PNF techniques. Before going into the stretch, push your forearm, elbow, and palm into the doorjamb, tightening your shoulder and pectoral areas, contracting the muscle and holding it for 10 seconds. Relax and go immediately into the stretch.

If you have tight shoulders, motion loss in your shoulders, or rotator cuff issues, consider the towel stretch alternative. Use a small towel held behind you. Use the towel to first pull your upper arm downward (improves external rotation) and then use the upper arm to pull the lower one upward (improves internal rotation). Alternate arms.

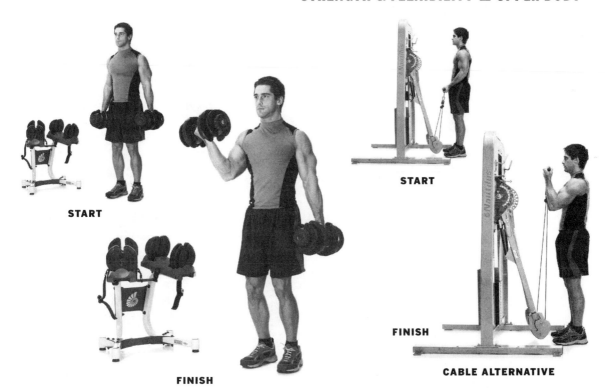

START

FINISH

START

FINISH

CABLE ALTERNATIVE

Biceps Curl

Curl weight up slowly, pausing at the top and letting the weight down slowly in a controlled motion. Don't arch your back to help (cheat) with the lift. With a dumbbell, start with the weights at your side, palms inward; as you get halfway up the lift, supinate slowly so your palm is facing upward at the end of the lift to better contract the biceps.

■ **Alternate biceps cable exercise:** A standing biceps curl with upper cable isolates your biceps nicely and helps develop your biceps "peak."

■ Free weights can include dumbbells or barbells. Curls can also be done while standing on tubing.

OrthoCheck

■ If you have lower back problems, try seated biceps curls with dumbbells.

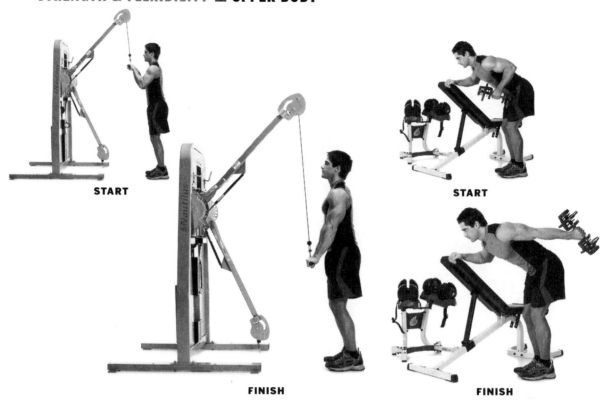

START

START

FINISH

FINISH

Triceps Extension

Move the weights slowly into full extension so you can squeeze and fully contract the triceps. Do not suddenly "lock out" your elbow, rather, slowly squeeze the motion until your elbows are straight.

■ Alternates include a one-arm dumbbell kickback supported on a bench, a rope pulley cable triceps extension, and an elastic tubing pulldown or kickback.

OrthoCheck

■ If you have elbow problems, especially pain behind the elbow when you fully straighten your arm, then resist the temptation to fully lock out your elbows.

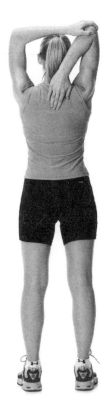

TriSho Stretch

To stretch the triceps and shoulder area as well as the upper lats, reach your right arm up and behind you, patting yourself on the upper back. Next use your left hand to grab your right elbow and gently pull your elbow in toward your head, allowing your right hand to reach further down your back over your left shoulder blade.

Hold for 10 seconds and switch sides.

■ **PNF alternative:** Before you start your stretch, while holding your right elbow with your left hand, with the elbow tip pointing upward, try to pull down your right elbow back toward your side but don't let it move, resisting the motion with your left hand.

Hold for 10 seconds, relax, and immediately go into the full TriSho Stretch.

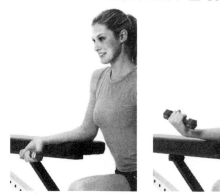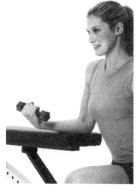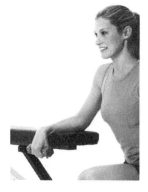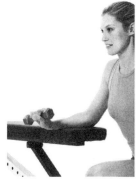

Forearm Strength

Forearm strengthening starts with a light dumbbell or elastic tubing. Perform wrist curls followed by reverse wrist curls.

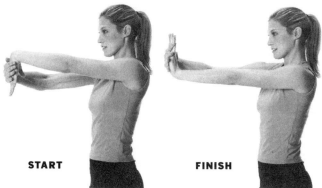

START   FINISH

Forearm Stretch

For wrist, forearm, and elbow flexibility, keep the left elbow straight in front of you. Let your wrist drop downward. Keeping your fingers straight, use your right hand to push downward on the top of your left hand until your wrist is flexed downward to a 90-degree angle. Hold for 10 seconds. Next, keeping your left elbow straight, extend your left wrist upward (Policeman's Stop). Use your right hand to simultaneously pull back both your fingers, thumb, and right palm at the same time so that your wrist is extended upward 90 degrees and your fingers are fully straight or even bent backward a little if possible. Alternate arms. Repeat each side again and then shake out both hands for a few seconds.

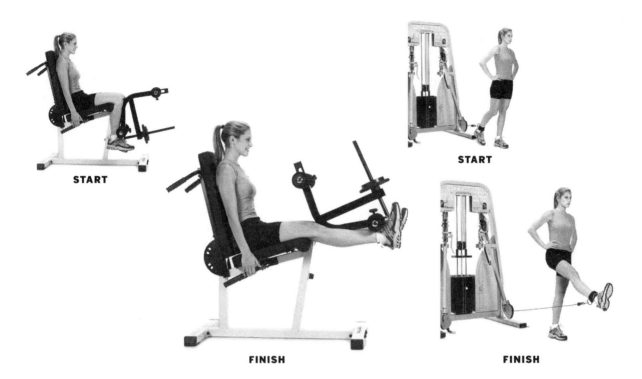

START

FINISH

START

FINISH

Leg Extension

Perform lift slowly, concentrating on tightening the quadriceps at the end of the movement.

■ **Modification:** If you have patellar problems, omit Leg Extension and follow the suggestions on Patellar Pain Syndrome on page 217. Also, you may be able to do a limited arc within your painfree range. Often patellar problems are in the midrange of the exercise so you can work the muscle in partial comfortable range. This includes pinning the weight stack out so that you are lifting only in the last 15 to 20 degrees of extension. This " short arc" version can be done either on a machine or even with ankle weights (see Concentration VMO "Short Arc" on page 122).

OrthoCheck

■ **Seat adjustment is important. Too far forward or backward puts undo pressure on the kneecap.**

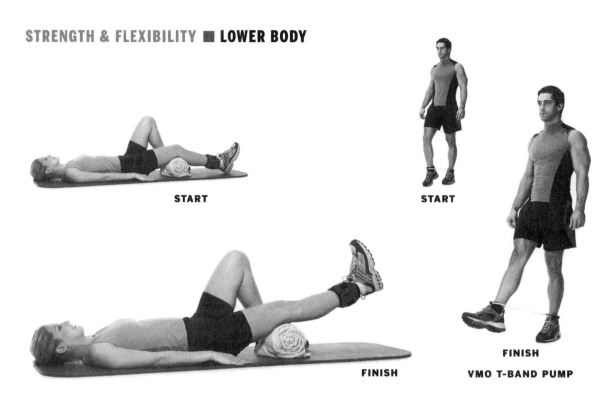

START

START

FINISH

FINISH

VMO T-BAND PUMP

Concentration VMO "Short Arc"

Lie on the floor with your left knee flexed and your left foot flat on the floor and your right leg straight out with a rolled towel under the knee. Using your quad (front thigh) muscle, lift your right heel off the ground, tightening the thigh until your right leg is fully straightened. Do not use the front of your hip to lift the leg off the towel. You should actually be slightly pressing back with your right knee to squeeze and flatten the towel. Feel your VMO (vastus medialis obliquus), the small muscle just above and towards the inner side of the kneecap, to make sure it is tight and stays tight for the 5 to 7 seconds you hold the leg straight. **Hold for 5 to 7 seconds and alternate legs.**

■ Another "short arc" version is the T-Band Pumps in which elastic tubing or a Theraband is tied around the ankles with your feet approximately shoulder-width. Turn the working leg outward slightly allowing the knee to slightly flex. Lift the foot off the ground and perform a pumping-action, thigh-tightening, knee-straightening exercise with the elastic as resistance.

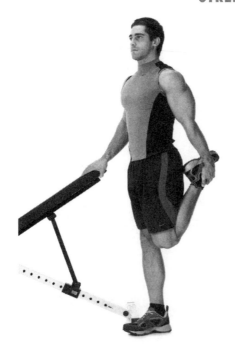

Quad Stretch

Stand straight but use your right hand to support you (until you get really good at this and can balance without difficulty). Grab your left foot with your left hand and bring your heel up to your buttock. Stand tall, don't lean forward at the waist or upper body.

Hold for 10 seconds and alternate sides.

Keep your knees together at all times, resisting the temptation to allow your thigh to move outward. The body cheats two ways to allow you to get your foot to your buttock, and you should avoid these cheats. In the first cheat, to get your foot to your buttock, spread your knees, abducting your hip. In the second cheat, you look downward and lean slightly forward, relaxing the front of your hip and upper quad. Both take away the effectiveness of the stretch.

■ **More advanced version:** If you can easily get your heel to your buttock, then increase the stretch by standing tall, keeping your knees inward and touching. Next pull back on your foot extending your hip backward while staying tall and not leaning forward. Your knee should be pointing backward slightly.

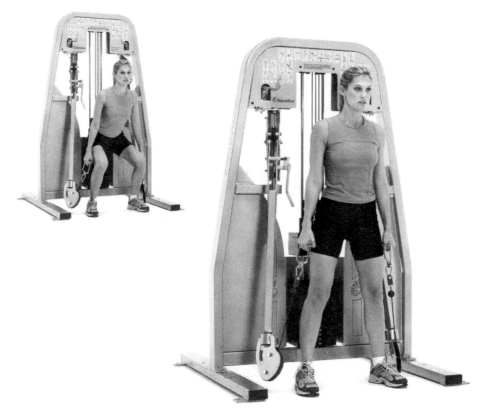

FREEDOM TRAINER START

Squat/Leg Press

Keep abdominals tight. Keep your weight on your heels, not your toes. Do not allow your thighs to go past parallel on the squat, although on the leg press machine you can go deeper as comfort allows. Do not bounce to get back up.

■ **Alternate:** If you are unable to perform squats or leg press because of patellar issues, see Patellar Pain Syndrome on page 217 and consider Horse, Partial Wall Seat, or Quad Isometrics (page 218), or "Short Arcs" (page 122) instead of this exercise.

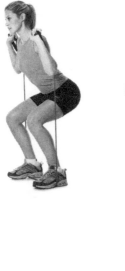

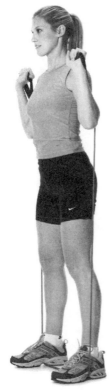

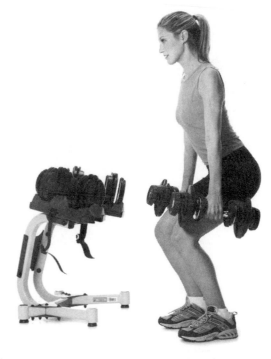

TUBING START

FREE WEIGHTS FINISH

ORTHOCHECK

■ If you have low back problems, use the Leg Press where you are more supported in a lying position rather than squats.

■ If you have patellar problems, use leg press, lighten weights and do higher reps (i.e., 20 to 25) and monitor for any increase in kneecap symptoms. Or, try quarter squats where instead of going down to parallel/90 degrees, you only drop down 25 percent within your comfort zone.

■ Also, if you have low back or patellar problems, start with the barbell only with squats and no weight added.

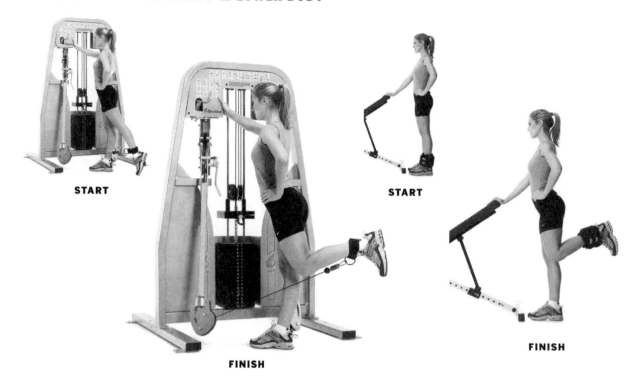

START

FINISH

START

FINISH

Leg Curls

Do not arch the back. Do not throw weight rapidly. Let weight back down slowly in a controlled manner.

■ **Alternates:** Try a standing kickback with tubing or ankle weights or standing leg curls with ankle weights.

OrthoCheck

■ **Do not look up, especially if you have neck problems. Rest your chin or forehead on the pad instead.**

■ **If you have lower back problems, move the weight even more slowly and resist the temptation to arch your back to complete the movement.**

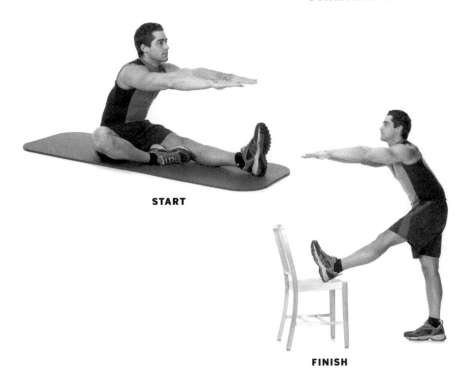

START

FINISH

Hamstring Stretch

Hamstrings are another problem area for many individuals. If you have tight hamstrings, low back problems, or have had hamstring pulls, then these should be performed daily.

Stay tall, don't hunch forward or lean forward.
Hold for 10 seconds, then alternate. Repeat each side again.

■ **Alternative:** Here is an easy version that can be done often at home: Start at the bottom of your staircase. Rest your right heel on one of the lower steps with your knee fully straight. Staying tall with arms out forward, lean into the staircase, feeling the stretch in your hamstring. Hold 10 to 20 seconds and alternate sides. As you get better, you can place your heel on higher steps. Remember, this is to be done at the bottom of the steps where it is safe.

■ **Hamstring PNF alternative:** So many individuals have difficulty with tight hamstrings, and often they need PNF techniques to regain flexibility. (See the hamstring PNF techniques on page 103.)

OrthoCheck

■ If you have lower back problems and find the seated hamstring stretch problematic, then try the standing version.

■ Also, if you have active sciatica with nerve irritation, including shooting pains down the entire leg, then avoid hamstring stretching until those nerve-related leg symptoms resolve. Some individuals have radiation into their buttock or thigh that is not true sciatica. Your physician or healthcare professional can help you decide whether it is time to start stretching your hamstrings. Eventually, hamstring stretches will be an important part of your low back health routine.

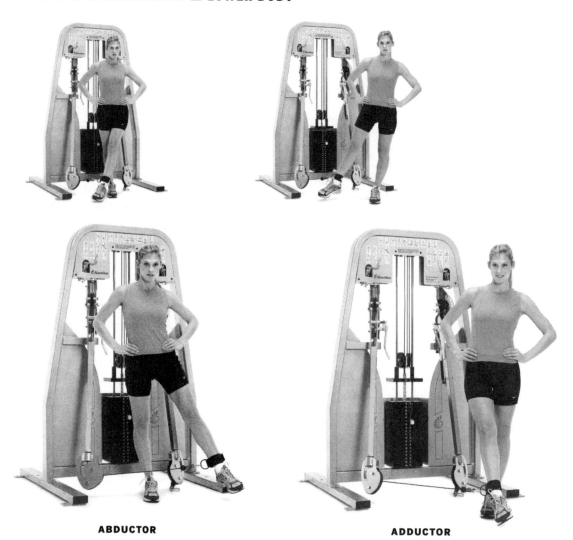

ABDUCTOR   ADDUCTOR

Hip Abductor and Adductor

Move weights slowly in a controlled manner. Do not bounce, especially when legs are wide apart and are being pulled back inward. Tighten abs during the movement.

■ **Alternate:** In addition to cable version, these can be done with ankle weights or elastic tubing and/or lower cable.

OrthoCheck

Movements should be controlled. Do not lean. If you have restricted hip movement, stay within your pain-free range of motion.

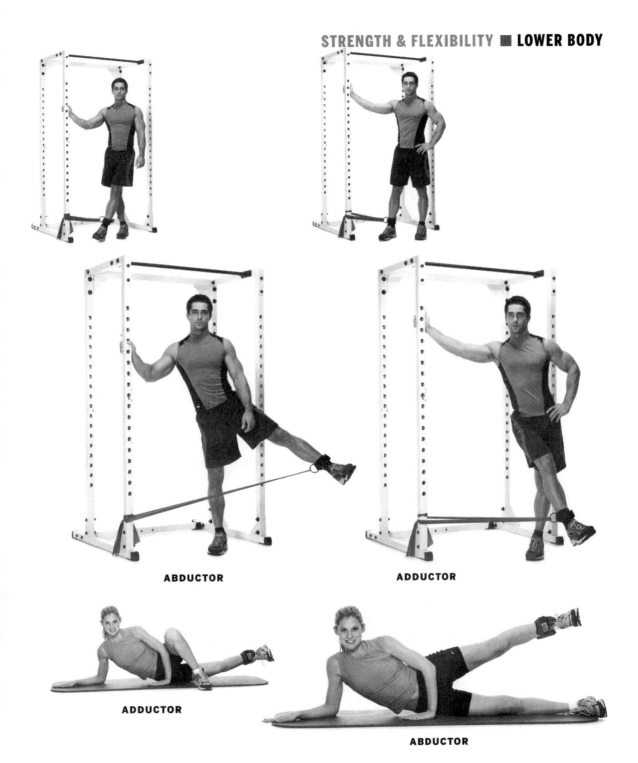

ABDUCTOR

ADDUCTOR

ADDUCTOR

ABDUCTOR

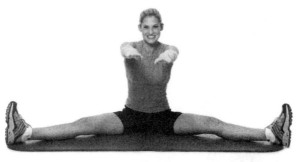

START

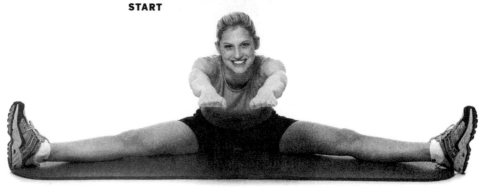

FINISH

Straddle Stretch

Good for the groin (adductor muscle) and hamstrings, this is also a great "partner stretch."

Hold for 10 seconds and alternate sides.

■ **Advanced:** An alternate more advanced version includes straddle with right and left bend.

■ **Modification:** Another home alternative includes using a staircase. Starting at the bottom of the steps, turn sideways so that your left leg is straight with the inner arch area of your left foot resting on one of the lower steps. Pick a step that gives you a slight stretching sensation on the inner thigh. While holding this position, allow your right knee to drop down slightly, enhancing the stretch on the left inner thigh.

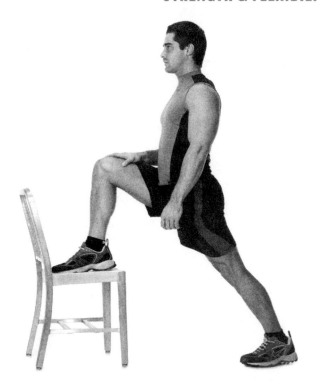

Psoas Stretch

To relieve hip and back pain

Place your right foot flat on the top of a chair, stool, or step approximately 2 feet high. Keep your left leg straight, foot pointing forward or slightly inward. Lean forward, keeping your back straight, until you feel a stretch in the front of your left hip.

Hold for 10 to 20 seconds and alternate sides.

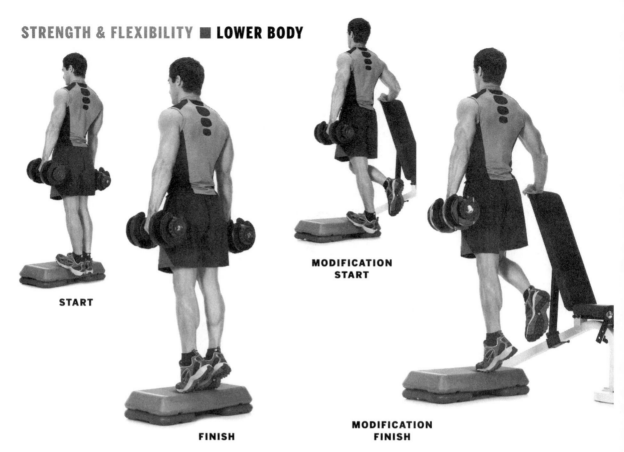

START

FINISH

MODIFICATION
START

MODIFICATION
FINISH

Calf Raise

Calf raises can be done using both legs at once or one at a time. With machines, I prefer both legs at once. When working off a step or flat ground, I prefer one leg at a time.

If you can do 20 calf raises on each side without weights, then start adding weights to either the machine or by holding dumbbells in your hands.

■ Calf raises can also be done on a leg press machine when using a lighter weight. Your legs are pressed outward and once in this position, use your ankles and calves to perform the lifting movement within that very short range.

■ Problems with residual calf weakness (both strength and endurance) follow many lower extremity injuries, from the foot up to hip.

ORTHOCHECK

■ If you have had any prior injuries, from the low back down, check your calf strength and endurance, including the "hop" test (page 52).

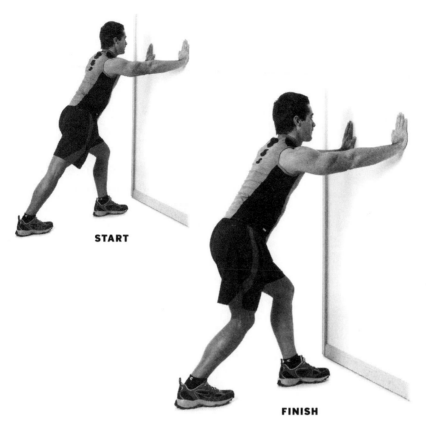

START

FINISH

Calf Stretch

This stretch is good for the gastrocnemius and soleus muscles, Achilles tendon and the plantar fascia (arch) area.

The calf muscle has two major components: the upper portion or gastrocnemius, (which actually crosses the back of the knee) and the soleus or lower portion, which becomes your Achilles tendon behind your ankle. The gastroc–soleus complex crosses two joints (knee and ankle), and because they are two separate muscles, they need to be stretched separately.

Start with your knee straight, stretching the soleus (hold 10 seconds), then bring your foot forward a little and do the flexed-knee version, which you will feel lower down (more for the soleus and Achilles tendon).

■ An alternate stretch can be done off a step or machine by allowing your heel to drop. Also, barefoot is better for calf stretching.

ORTHOCHECK

■ Keep your foot pointed straight ahead or preferably even "pigeon-toed" inward a little. The cheat or mistake is to turn your foot outward a little, which allows your foot to roll a little into pronation, making this stretch easier, and thus less effective.

"A" R & R (ACTIVE REST AND RECOVERY)

A bow that is stretched
to its fullest capacity
may certainly snap.
A sword that is tempered
to its very sharpest
may easily be broken.

LAO TSU, IN THE TAO TE CHING

YOUR BODY NEEDS to recover, not just when it's been injured, but every time you've had a serious workout. Your tissues need downtime between bouts of exercise in order to engage in the repair and remodeling I discussed in Chapter 2. Chris Carmichael, Lance Armstrong's coach says, "We treat recovery as a scheduled workout."

So, a hot tub or massage and a good night's sleep?

That shouldn't be a hard sell, right?

Unfortunately, many people who exercise are puritanical about it. They seem to think that if they're not constantly pushing themselves and punishing themselves, then they must be getting soft. In reality, the genuine gains in fitness happen while you're at rest, and they often show up in performance after you've had a little time off.

In 1954, a young athlete and medical student named Roger Bannister took 5 days off from his training, then ran the world's first sub-4-minute mile. There are countless stories of swimmers who get the flu, miss several days of training, then come back in the water and have their personal best times. These athletes always had the skills; they simply needed a metabolic recovery in order to do their best.

KNOW YOUR LIMITS

We admire athletes who put their bodies on the line when the big game is at stake, but the rest of us need to be a bit more reasonable and know when discretion is the greater part of valor.

More is not always better. Pushing harder all of the time will bring you to a point of diminishing returns, where gains turn to losses. For an elite athlete, the result could be a 1 to 2 percent drop in performance, or worse, an injury. That's the difference between making the Olympic team and staying home. For the rest of us, it means that our exercise plan starts to backfire and becomes counterproductive. We don't quite feel as good, or we're sidelined with an injury.

Problems can happen gradually over time with nagging overuse injuries or overtraining syndrome, or they can be more sudden or dramatic. When you push your body to the breaking point, something often gives way. I seem to get far more calls from athletes needing help whenever the competition heats up, whether it's a regional ice-skating tournament or the Olympic Trials. The race between adaptation and metabolic overload or injury often leaves a body count, and the decisive factor in that race is usually the rest and recovery (R&R).

Simple fatigue increases the likelihood of injury. Being tired diminishes the precision of motor control and interrupts voluntary muscle-stabilizing activity. Ask anybody in the ski industry—or any orthopaedist, for that matter—and they'll tell you that injuries on the slopes are highest in the afternoon. In football, most injuries are in the third quarter. Heavy exercise has been shown to even cause a (temporary) decline in cognitive function. Another culprit, especially with regard to knee injuries, seems to be a decline in proprioception—body awareness that affects balance and coordination—and neuromuscular control in the lower extremities.

Bottom line: Rest and recovery are essential elements in any exercise program that is going to do more good than harm.

When you train your body, you tax it in a variety of ways. This includes both local and systemic overload. Work your biceps, and you're loading that entire complex of muscles and tendons. Overwork it with inadequate rest between workouts, and you get sore and actually start losing biceps strength. Run everyday, and you are pounding leg bones and joints. Do it right, and your bones (and other supporting structures) get stronger; overdo it, and you have a tibial stress fracture.

These local responses happen wherever you specifically train. In addition to the local effects, though, there is also a systemic or metabolic cost to exercise. All that you do,

■ ■ ■ OVERTRAINING SYNDROME

The following signs and symptoms are indicative of overtraining syndrome:

■ Prolonged recovery from workouts
■ Persistent muscle soreness and stiffness
■ Drop in performance
■ Fatigue
■ Altered mood (i.e., depression, irritability)
■ Loss of drive
■ Loss of appetite
■ Elevated pulse rate in the morning resting heart rate
■ Overuse injuries

With weight training, never work the same muscle group 2 days in a row. Most individuals need 2 to 3 days for adequate muscle recovery after a good upper or lower body workout.

Never run 2 days in a row, but that doesn't mean you can't do aerobics every day. Mixing up your mode—swimming, biking, skipping rope—distributes the stresses around the body in a more productive, less destructive way.

Core work can be done every other day or even daily in some instances, especially if you're not working to the max. Rehab exercises, usually involving less intensity and thus less stress and strain on the involved muscles, usually need to be done daily (or even numerous times a day) to stimulate early recovery and gains.

Walking, stretching, yoga, and other light workouts, as well as rehabilitation exercises, can and should be done every day.

But even when you're cross-training, it all adds up in terms of metabolic cost to the system as a whole, so plan 1 day off a week.

Also, follow the 10 percent rule: Never increase your workouts (i.e., amount lifted or miles run) more than 10 percent per week. This allows the time you need for necessary adaptation. The 10 percent rule especially applies when you're coming off an injury and the desire to make up for lost time can toss you back on the injured reserve list all too often.

especially in direct proportion to the intensity, duration, and frequency of your activities, taxes your entire body.

Even if you vary the activities and body parts involved, there is a cumulative toll on the system as a whole, with local and systemic stresses adding up. It is easy to see how even seemingly good workout programs can get you into trouble with overtraining. The result is systemic breakdown (system crash) or local breakdown with acute or overuse injury.

Your morning resting heart rate (MRHR) can be a barometer of overtraining syndrome along with other signs and symptoms. Get used to taking your resting heart rate in the morning before getting out of bed. Monitor it daily upon awakening, especially in times of heavier training. As you become more fit, your heart rate should gradually lower. If your MRHR increases more than 5 beats per minute, that is a sign that you may be overtraining, not allowing for adequate recovery between workouts.

SNOOZE, DON'T LOSE

It's during sleep that you maximize recovery and growth. Getting plenty of sleep isn't a sign of laziness; it's a vital part of keeping fit.

Sleep deprivation can lead to circulatory problems, weight gain, and hormonal imbalances, as well as an inability to process carbohydrates and manage stress. Sleeplessness increases the levels of cortisol in your blood, which encourages insulin resistance.

Studies show that men and women who sleep less than 6 hours, or more than 9 hours, have higher mortality rates and higher rates of cancer and heart disease. Also, if you sleep 10 hours or more a night, you begin to lose bone density.

Studies abound showing a variety of ways in which inadequate sleep impairs mental function—from basic alertness to complex problem solving. We all need sleep to convert short-term memories—the day's events—into long-term memory.

While we sleep, our minds work through the problems that baffled us during the day. And yet, according to the Report of the National Commission on Sleep Disorders Research, 40 million North Americans experience chronic sleep and wakefulness disorders.

To improve your sleep:

- Make sure your bedroom is completely dark, or wear eye shades

- Keep your sleeping space and your working space separate (In other words, don't put your desk in your bedroom.)

- Read just before bed—don't watch TV

- Don't have caffeine after lunch

- Invest in a good, comfortable mattress

If you need a sleep aid, first try boosting your diet with 5-hydroxtryptophan (5-HTP) to increase serotonin production in the central nervous system. Supplements of melatonin, a substance that occurs naturally in your body, can help get you back on track with better sleep patterns, especially with travel-related (time zone change) sleep difficulties and jet lag. You shouldn't use this supplement for more than a day or two.

Calcium and magnesium are two minerals that are essential for proper relaxation, and some individuals feel that magnesium taken at bedtime can help with sleep.

We know that low magnesium levels can increase your need for oxygen during exercise, resulting in quicker muscle fatigue. Valerian (*Valeriana officinalis*) is a supplement than can be used on a temporary basis to promote relaxation and improve sleep. Like melatonin, it is not a long-term solution for ongoing sleep difficulties, which should be discussed with your physician. If you have a sleep problem that persists, visit a sleep lab at a hospital near you that offers testing that can get to the root of your problem.

BREAK UP THE ROUTINE AND CLEANSE THE SYSTEM

Cross-training allows you to rest certain muscle groups while working on others, but even with a well-balanced exercise routine that isn't overtaxing any particular joints or muscle groups, metabolic waste is added to your system.

Distance runners, for instance, use oxygen at 100 to 200 times the normal rate, which can lead to a buildup of free radicals, the extremely reactive form of oxygen associated with cell damage and implicated in some cancers. Intense exercise also depletes vitamin E, one of the body's prime defenders against oxidative stress. Exercise can also damage lipids, fatty substances that are an important part of cell structure and serve as fuel.

This is why blood flow to cleanse the system is so important, and that's where a light swim or bike ride, Tai Chi, or that hot tub or massage comes in. These techniques aren't just a hedonistic indulgence. Rhythmic circulatory activity creates a "flush and fuel" environment for your muscles and organs, especially when combined with eating plenty of antioxidant-rich fruits and veggies, along with proper carbohydrate intake, as discussed in Step 6 on page 142.

THE DIFFERENCE BETWEEN GOOD PAIN AND BAD PAIN

When you "feel the burn" during a workout, you're experiencing immediate muscle soreness (IMS), caused by the buildup of lactic acid and other metabolic wastes in the muscles. There's no harm in this. It's one of the side effects of a really productive workout, and this "good pain" will go away shortly after exercise.

The time to worry is when you feel sensations like stinging, stabbing, sharp pain, or tingling numbness instead of a healthy burn. Stop what you're doing. Muscle may burn a little, but joints shouldn't. These sensations could be signs of a muscle tear, a tendon strain, or ligament strain. If you're in a gym, a trainer may be able to tell you what went wrong. But if the pain persists, see your doctor.

With time you will get pretty good at telling the difference between good pain and bad pain. In caring for pro athletes, every day we have to make the call to determine whether or not an athlete can still play with an injury. This comes down to knowing the difference between hurt and harm. If the injury is relatively minor, it may hurt a little, but there will be no harm to the athlete in competing. For those, we give the athlete a green light or flashing yellow light and monitor him or her. Other injuries might not even hurt too much, but we know that they are inherently more dangerous with the potential for either short-term or long-term harm. For them it's a red light. Playing is simply not worth the risk.

The pain or discomfort in muscles that have undergone unaccustomed vigorous exercise, particularly involving eccentric muscle contractions, is commonly called delayed-onset muscle soreness or DOMS. There's tenderness and stiffness, but not the classic inflammatory response, and a stronger sensation than the "burning" experienced during and immediately following maximal exercise. The soreness is thought to come from microscopic tears to the muscle fibers that occur primarily during eccentric or "negative" exercise, which means the muscle is lengthening or elongating while producing force. That burn is also from metabolic processes producing lactic acid and other noxious substances that accumulate in exercising muscle.

Typically, the soreness begins a few hours after exercise. It becomes most prominent 12 to 48 hours afterward and continues for several days regardless of whether there is further activity. It usually responds to rest and nonsteroidal anti-inflammatory drugs (NSAIDs). Light massage and stretching helps, as does a very light rhythmic aerobic exercise (like stationary cycling) to get blood flowing through the involved muscles, which helps clear the metabolic waste products. Delayed-onset muscle soreness is not cause for alarm, but it deserves attention.

To avoid DOMS, take it slow and easy. Your body needs time to build up to tolerating certain loads. If you engage in heavier, "negative" workouts as an advanced training aid, expect more soreness and allow more recovery time.

Go easy on the ibuprofen (Advil and Motrin), which may not be the best choice in dealing with the pain of muscle soreness. Aspirin and ibuprofen block the production of prostaglandin, which stimulates muscle repair and is associated with pain during recovery. Ointments like Icy Hot and Tiger Balm may help and give a sensation of relief, but they do it by irritating the skin, producing sensations of heat or cold that temporarily mask the pain of the sore muscle. In truth, the rubbing may actually be what helps when you apply a balm or cream.

Other aids include "The Stick," a device that allows for excellent self-massage of sore muscles can be helpful. Electrical stimulation devices, like H-Wave are used by athletes worldwide to enhance muscle recovery and decrease muscle soreness.

Eat soy and other antioxidants. As I'll explain more fully in Step 6, the isoflavones found in soy protein produce antioxidant effects, which may help reduce soreness and inflammation. Also, studies have shown that increasing your fruit and vegetable consumption (to 6 to 9 servings a day) will significantly reduce oxidative damage. Antioxidant supplements are thought to help, too, but nothing beats the real deal, which comes from the produce department of your local supermarket.

Keep moving. You'd think that complete rest would be the best remedy for soreness, but in reality, light exercise can help.

WATCH OUT FOR OVERTRAINING

Some level of burnout is natural after a steady slog of hard work. Even 8 weeks after a marathon, a runners' muscles are still regenerating, trying to recover, and their immune systems are depleted, making them more prone to colds and the flu. Again, exercise is medicine with a dose-response curve. Exercise a little and you boost your immunity, or overdose and it's depleted.

Simple "overreaching" leads to muscle soreness, decreased coordination, dampened libido, and often times, more frequent colds and coughs. What we call "tapering," a period of lighter training, will usually cure this.

Persistent underperforming, with or without the depression or anxiety of overreaching, that does not respond to 2 weeks of tapering or rest, may be true overtraining. This combination of psychological stress and inadequate recovery time can cause immunosuppression, hormonal imbalances, and chronic inflammation. Other symptoms include lethargy, boredom, nagging muscle soreness, and a marked increase in your resting heart rate.

Ten to 20 percent of all athletes and 60 percent of elite distance runners fall into overtraining at least once in their careers. Most often, athletes overtrain when they adopt the regime of a famous star, train without a coach or partner, or train with athletes at a much higher level.

Athletes and active individuals on the low-carb bandwagon are particularly susceptible to the overtraining blahs. Inadequate fluid intake will also get you into trouble pretty quickly.

INJURY AND REST

One of the trickiest things about being injured is getting the balance right between continued activity, which can make the injury worse, and complete inactivity, which can lead to stiffness or other problems. One problem includes deconditioning, meaning that the gains you've worked so hard to achieve slip away.

Serious athletes usually can't tolerate complete rest, so we put them on "therapeutic exercise," usually for 6 to 8 weeks. This means lighter aerobic exercise that avoids the athlete's usual activities. Runner's swim, swimmer's bike, and so on. Of course, these elite performers have to resist the temptation to compete and improve. Sometimes, the lack of a killer workout gets them down psychologically, but that's where massage and whirlpool come in handy, for stress relief as well as for soothing soreness and improving circulation. Allowing athletes to remain active and fit, in a safe manner, while their injuries heal, helps psychologically. And when you're exercising to rehabilitate, the demands for recovery time are far less than when you are working a muscle to exhaustion. You can do light, rehab exercises a couple of times a day, everyday.

BOUNCING BACK

One thing's for sure—trying to make up for lost time by rebounding with a vengeance is the best way to put yourself back on the sideline far worse off than before. This is all too common with individuals coming off an injury. They ramp up too quickly.

Our friend Jose Reyes, the Mets second baseman, struggled with his hamstring throughout the spring of 2004, largely because he tried to come back too soon. It flared up again, they did an MRI, and they found that, after almost 7 weeks of rehabilitation, his hamstring had not healed.

San Diego Padres outfielder Jay Payton, who had multiple hamstring strains with the Mets in 2001, put it this way, "When you think you're ready, take another week off."

AVOID "BETTER LIVING THROUGH CHEMISTRY"

Performance-enhancing substances are hidden in training rooms and lockers everywhere, because everyone is looking for an edge. Years ago the medical and scientific communities said that anabolic steroids do not work, but they do. When you combine anabolic steroids with a proper workout and nutrition, you do get size. You flip the switch for muscle protein growth, you shed body fat, and you get a quicker recovery after hard workouts.

It all sounds too good to be true. Of course, it is too good to be true.

Anabolic steroids wreak havoc on your body systems with many short-term and long-term side effects, some permanent. They are especially dangerous in growing children, yet studies have estimated that 10 to 12 percent of high school males have experimented with them.

Anabolic steroids also damage your frame. They may give you bigger muscles, but they actually weaken the tendons and muscle-tendon junctions that anchor these big muscles to your bones. This is one of the reasons I see big strong individuals "blowing out" their pecs or quads and winding up on the operating room table. Steroids are a really stupid move. They are not worth the price you pay. Period. The FrameWork way will get you where you need to be. It just takes a bit more patience and persistence.

YOU ARE WHAT YOU JUST ATE (FUELING A HEALTHY FRAME)

MARTINA NAVRATILOVA, an athlete clearly built to last, says, "When it comes to what you eat, what you put in is what you get out."

Nutrition—good or bad—not only affects your heart, your skin, your susceptibility to certain diseases, and your waistline, it also has a direct impact on your frame. As we discussed in Chapter 3, your body has an amazing capacity for self-repair, but you won't help the cause by stuffing yourself with potato chips and Dr Pepper. The ongoing remodeling of bones, muscles, joints, tendons, and ligaments requires the right kind of fuel. And exercise itself actually increases the body's nutritional demands, making it all the more important that when you refuel, you do it at the premium pump.

Working out accelerates the body's catabolic activity (the tearing down of cells), at the same time that it accelerates the body's anabolic properties (the building back up). By making you sweat, exercise drains the body of vital moisture that needs to be replenished. The increased burning of oxygen driven by exercise—oxidation—produces free radicals, the chemical wild cards that seek to bond randomly with other molecules, and in so doing disrupt normal cell growth and metabolism. Free radicals are implicated in certain cancers, but when these monkey wrenches pinball through your cells, they also do damage to muscles, tendons, and joints.

It's also true that certain nutrients most of us consume every day can make inflammation worse, block metabolism of calcium in your bones, add to the drying out of your cells, and add pounds of excess baggage—fat—for your frame to have to carry around.

On the other hand, simply by eating right, you can actually:

■ Reduce the inflammation in the "itis" conditions such as tendonitis, bursitis, arthritis, and synovitis

■ Enhance tissue repair and remodeling in joints, tendons, muscles, and ligaments, especially after injury

■ Add moisture to your cells and lubrication for your joints

■ Provide the enzymes necessary for proper cell growth and function

■ Provide antioxidants to offset free radicals

■ Provide vital minerals such as calcium and enhance their metabolism

A DIET FOR HEALTHY BONES AND JOINTS

As an active person, you need to realize that food and drink aren't just a matter of responding to hunger and thirst, and eating a proper diet isn't just about controlling your weight. Nutrition, like exercise, is a form of medicine.

To get the nutrition that will heal and sustain your frame, you need to follow a diet rich in protein, balanced with the right type and amount of carbohydrates and fats, supplemented with multivitamins and especially antioxidants, and all washed down with a lot more water than you think you need.

What is it that athletes and active individuals need for a solid, durable frame?

CARBOHYDRATES

Yes, a great many Americans need to lose some weight, and a good many are relying on the high protein, low carb diets that are all the rage.

But carbohydrates are our best source of energy, and this is especially true for athletes. The American Dietetic Association and the American College of Sports Medicine recommend that 55 to 58 percent of your calories come from carbohydrates, 12 to 15 percent come from protein, and 25 to 30 percent from fat, though the total amount of carbohydrates will vary day to day depending on whether you jog a little or run a lot. In general, I recommend a four to one ratio of carbs to protein.

And if eating carbs for health sounds like heresy, remember that it's excess calories that make you fat, not carbohydrates. Studies at Yale and Stanford published in the *Journal of the American Medical Association* show that weight loss on low carb diets comes primarily from lower caloric intake, not from lower carbs per se. Another study at Tufts-New England Medical Center in Boston compared the Atkins, Ornish, Weight Watchers, and Zone diets and found them all similar in their results. Those who lost the most ate the least calories—simple as that.

Nature provided carbohydrates for a reason. People who cut out the carbs often don't eat enough fruits and vegetables, which you need for many reasons, not the least of which is that they provide antioxidants that every active person needs to ward off cell damage.

The proper balance of carbs and protein is how we maintain glycogen in the muscles and in the liver. If your carbs are low, your glycogen will be low, which encourages your body to break down the protein in muscle to obtain energy, which makes you more prone to injury.

The glycemic index (GI) teaches us that "all carbs are not created equal" in terms of the effect on our metabolic systems, both short and long term. The GI ranks foods from 1 to 100 based on how rapidly the carbs enter your system or your bloodstream. Foods with a GI over 60 are considered fast and give you rapid energy. Those under 40 are slower and are more useful for recovery.

Where a food ranks on the GI tells us nothing about its overall nutritional value. Soda, for example, has an extremely high GI but no value other than that it's a liquid. And foods ranked either high and low on the index can benefit athletes depending on the timing. Endurance athletes do better if they consume a low GI meal 1 to 4 hours before the event; higher GI meals are better for muscle recovery afterward, because they refuel the cells more quickly.

But the downside of high GI foods is that some of the insulin surge they provide goes directly into fat cells for long-term storage. The more highly refined the carb—the highest being such things as white sugar and white bread—the faster they burn, giving you a sudden rush, followed by that empty feeling. Believe it or not, most of us consume 50 percent of our carbs as these simple sugars. So our insulin levels are yo-yoing up and down, and our fat cells are packing it away. That's why the best carbs are the ones in whole grains, fruits, and vegetables, where the fiber slows down the absorption of nutrients into a steady flow.

Lack of carbohydrates makes athletes irritable and exhausted and knocks them off their game. During serious endurance exercise, you need 30 to 60 grams of carbohydrate each hour to maintain blood-glucose levels and to replace muscle glycogen. You should eat at least 200 grams 3 to 4 hours before higher-intensity exercise, or up to 100 grams an hour before. After exercise you need 6 grams of carb per pound of body weight every 2 to 4 hours for up to 6 hours.

The best way to eat your carbs is with small amounts of protein to enhance uptake into the muscles, especially during the recovery phase after your workout.

PROTEIN

While carbs replace glycogen, protein after exercise restores the amino acids you need to repair muscles. Various studies have shown that the sooner after exercise you eat the protein, the better for your physiological recovery. If you can tolerate it, the best time for eating the protein you'll need for muscle recovery is actually before you exert yourself.

Protein needs vary depending on your activity level and the intensity of your workout, but it's usually between 12 to 15 percent of your daily total calories or sometimes as high as 20 percent in certain instances. Endurance athletes need 1.2 to 1.4 g/kg of body weight of protein per day, whereas weight lifters may

need 1.6 to 1.8 g/kg. But in either case, it's possible to obtain this through your diet. Sedentary individuals in comparison need only 0.8 g/kg. Lean and red meats are packed with protein and also give you plenty of iron and zinc. Vegetarians sometimes get into trouble because of their lack of protein, but this is not necessary if they consume plenty of soy, vegetables, and eggs.

FAT

In our svelte-conscious society, most of us think of fat as a form of toxic waste. However, you need fat for insulation, for hormone production, to maintain your cell membrane structure, to metabolize fat-soluble vitamins, and for endurance in exercise.

Fat provides twice the calories per gram as carbohydrates or protein, which is why weight-watching Americans wisely try to avoid it. But in studies of differing fat content in diets with the same total calories, the people who consumed a moderate amount of fat performed 14 percent better in endurance than the low-fat group.

The minimal level of body fat for health is 5 percent for males and 12 percent for females. While the American Dietetic Association recommends a diet of 25 to 30 percent fat, and, even though it sounds like heresy, you should consume 20 to 30 percent of your calories as fat, the average American consumes over 40 percent of their calories in fats! Even so, it's the type of fat we eat that's the problem, not the fat per se. Other parts of the problem include the size of the portions and the amount of food that is highly processed and sugary.

Seventy to 80 percent of your fats should come from the mono- or polyunsaturated variety.

The bad fats you want to avoid are saturated, meaning that they have as many hydrogen molecules as possible. These are butter, margarine, and other animal fats. They congeal at room temperature, which gives you some idea what they do in your coronary arteries.

These fats affect the way we make prostaglandins, the hormones that regulate inflammation. A meal high in saturated fat increases the inflammatory proteins associated with heart disease, and this elevated level can last for 3 or 4 hours. Inflammation also negatively affects your musculoskeletal tissues in dozens of ways.

The very worst fats are the partially hydrogenated or hydrogenated fats, also known as trans fats, created when hydrogen has been added to vegetable oil to increase the shelf life and flavor stability of foods such as cookies, crackers, and margarine. Trans fats lower the "good" cholesterol (high-density lipoprotein, or HDL) and increase the "bad" cholesterol (low-density lipoprotein, or LDL). They make the arteries more rigid, cause them to clog, and contribute to type 2 diabetes. So what's good for shelf life is very bad for your life.

The monounsaturated fats (so called because they have one double chemical bond) found in avocados, olive oil, peanut oil, flaxseed oil, and canola oil are actually good for you. They can even help you burn off stored body fat. In a 30-week study, people eating peanuts actually lowered their blood

levels of triglycerides, the chemical form fat takes en route to your fat cells.

Even more beneficial are the polyunsaturated fats (meaning that they have two or more double bonds). These are linoleic and linolenic acid, also known as omega-6 and omega-3 fatty acids. We call these "essential fatty acids," not just because we need them, but because our bodies don't produce them. They have to be part of our diet.

The essential fatty acids are vital for maintaining a healthy frame, and they can be a major boost for individuals troubled by arthritis, tendinitis, and other joint problems.

We normally get plenty of omega-6 (linoleic) in what we eat. It's found in all vegetable oils, such as safflower, sunflower, and corn oils, most grains and beans, as well as poultry and eggs.

The one we need to eat more of is omega-3 (linolenic). Omega-3 is a natural lubricant for the articular surfaces of your joints, as well as for other gliding surfaces such as tendons and bursae. It's found primarily in cold-water fish—salmon, sardines, mackerel—but one type is found in dark green leafy vegetables, as well as in flaxseed oil, pumpkin, soy and canola oil, and walnuts. Wild game such as venison and buffalo are also good sources of omega-3s.

The health benefits of omega-3 first came to light in the 1970s, when scientists studying the Inuits of Greenland found that those native people suffered far less from coronary heart disease, arthritis, diabetes mellitus, and psoriasis than did Europeans, even though their diet was loaded in fat. Eventually, researchers realized it was the omega-3s that gave the Inuits protection from these "diseases of affluence."

Many studies have shown participants with inflammatory diseases reporting less joint stiffness, swelling, tenderness, and overall fatigue when taking omega-3s. Research also shows that getting more omega-3 fatty acids enables some participants to reduce their use of nonsteroidal anti-inflammatory drugs (NSAIDs).

The typical American diet has about a 20 to 1 ratio of omega-6 to omega-3 fatty acids, but a one-to-one balance is the ideal.

Improving that balance means replacing vegetable oils—safflower, sunflower, corn—with olive oil. This is especially important if you have any form of inflammation, including aching joints.

Barring a move to Greenland to live off whale blubber, the best way to get more omega-3 is to eat Atlantic salmon and other fatty, preferably coldwater fish, including herring, sardines, Atlantic halibut, bluefish, tuna, and Atlantic mackerel. The American Heart Association recommends that people eat tuna or salmon at least twice a week, although tuna increases concern about consuming mercury. As an alternative, you can supplement your diet with fish-oil capsules containing omega-3s. I recommend ProCaps Omega-3 from Andrew Lessman's Your Vitamin line (www.yourvitamins.com).

WATER

Water is our most critical nutrient. It's the only one we can't do without for more than a few days. Your blood is 90 percent water. Your brain is 85 percent water, muscle is 72 percent, skin is 71 percent, bone is 30 percent, and fat is 15 percent water.

You need to drink 8 glasses (2 quarts) of water a day just to provide the cellular moisture you need and to help your kidneys filter your blood. When you exercise, you need substantially more fluid intake to balance your fluid loss. That means 14 to 22 ounces 2 hours before exercise and 6 to 12 ounces every 12 to 15 minute depending on your tolerance.

A study from the Gatorade Sports Science Institute in Barrington, Illinois, showed that a well-hydrated person has the capacity to exercise 33 percent longer than someone who is not. And yet the same study showed that half of exercisers are dehydrated before they even begin.

Gatorade and other sports drinks can be helpful, especially when you're engaged in a sustained workout for more than an hour. These drinks provide electrolytes that aid muscle contraction and carbohydrates that help retain liquid and stave off low blood glucose levels. But what you really need, first and foremost, is simple H_2O.

Water is a solvent for vitamins and minerals, and it transports these throughout your body. Water assists in muscle contraction. It makes digestion possible, serves as a shock absorber in everything from bone and muscle and connective tissue to your eyeballs, maintains your body temperature as it eliminates heat, and rids the body of wastes. So when you don't get enough water, everything dries out and nothing functions as well as it should.

As your body loses water, the effect registers first in those areas where you have the highest water content—blood, brain, muscle, and skin. This means that you lose mental ability, and you get weak muscles. If you watch a lot of sports, you've probably seen more than one extremely fit, elite athlete drop to the floor with severe muscle cramps brought on by even mild dehydration. Likewise, muscle pulls and other injuries are much more likely when you're dry.

When you feel beat—headache, sore muscles in your neck and back, eyestrain—it's not necessarily stress or that you need a vacation in Aruba. You may just need more water! And don't think that coffee or a Coke is going to perk you up. Caffeine, like alcohol, is a diuretic, meaning that it pulls more liquid out of the system than it adds. Less water in the system results in more mental fatigue and more of that draggy feeling. Keep in mind, too, that air travel and air conditioning both contribute to dehydration.

So a word to the wise: Don't wait till you are parched. Assume you're thirsty. When it doubt . . . drink water. When you're bored and need a break . . . take a drink of water. When you sit down for a meal . . . take a drink of water. As a marathon-running doctor friend of mine says, you want to be able to "pee clear." (But drink most of this liquid before 5 in the afternoon so you won't be up all night going to the bathroom.)

The water you need for your Monday morning workout, you have to drink on Sunday. If you exercise at the end of the day, top off with a couple of glasses of water 2 to 3 hours before exercise. In other words, "camel up."

Drinking plenty of water also helps with weight loss. It fills you up, cleanses your taste buds, and neutralizes food cravings.

And don't think that you have to buy bottled water. It isn't always any purer than tap, so go by taste. If it helps you drink more water to pay 2 bucks for it in a nifty little bottle, do it!

CALCIUM

Certain nutrients are absolutely essential for a healthy frame, and, thanks to the American Dairy Association (and maybe your mom), you can probably guess what's first on the list. After listening to years of advertising, anyone within earshot of radio or television will associate calcium with strong bones. And this is not a misperception. Calcium deficit is an invitation to stress fractures and other broken bones.

The other issue that has gained lots of attention is the loss of bone density in older women. Osteoporosis—the weakening of bone—affects one of every three postmenopausal woman, but it also affects men, as well as young women. Bone mass for everyone peaks at about age 30 and then declines. The focus has been on women because around menopause, significant bone loss can occur. The real take home message for everyone, young or old, man or woman, is that we need to store up healthy bone to be drawn on later, the same way you put away money in a savings account.

The truly critical period for strengthening

bone is the teen years. I've already described the butter-soft bones I've found in many female athletes coming in for surgery. The primary culprit is not enough calcium. Eighty percent of girls and 50 percent of boys aged 9 to 19 do not get the recommended 1,300 milligrams per day of calcium. But another villain is too much soda! It's not just that soda takes the place of milk. The phosphoric acid in soda actually interferes with the absorption of calcium into bones. The too little calcium being consumed is actually blocked from entering the system—a double whammy!

We also need to keep in mind that excessive alcohol decreases the absorption of calcium into the bones, and, as is the case with cigarettes, alcohol contains chemicals that are toxic to the cells that produce bone. High sodium (salt) has a negative effect on bone integrity, and more than two cups of coffee daily also can contribute to bone loss.

The minimum daily requirements for calcium are:

Children (4–8 years)	**800 mg**
Teenagers (9–18 years)	**1,300 mg**
Adults (19–50)	**1,000 mg**
Pregnant or nursing women	**1,200 mg**
Adults (51 or older)	**1,200 mg**
Postmenopausal women	**1,200–1,500 mg**

The body can absorb about 550 milligrams of calcium at one time. An 8-ounce glass of milk contains about 300 milligrams; two slices of firm cheese, such as American, Swiss, cheddar or mozzarella, have about the same.

Softer cheeses, like cottage cheese, most often contain a third to half of this amount.

Some stars in terms of delivering calcium are:

Yogurt (1 cup plain, 2 percent)	**415 mg**
Nonfat dry milk (¼ cup)	**377 mg**
Rhubarb (1 cup)	**348 mg**
Skim milk (1 cup)	**285 mg**
Salmon (3 to 4 ounces)	**225 mg**
Kale (1 cup)	**179 mg**
Beet greens (1 cup)	**165 mg**
Tofu (3 ounces)	**150 mg**
Almonds (3 ounces)	**150 mg**

Also, many foods such as orange juice and soy milk, as well as cereals like Total, come in calcium-fortified forms.

Calcium supplements are another safe way to get the calcium you need. The amount of calcium in supplements varies from 200 milligrams to 600 milligrams, so check the label, and also note that while a supplement "serving" may contain 400 milligrams of calcium, that "serving" may be two tablets. Calcium supplements are best absorbed when taken in doses of 500 milligrams or less, so this means that you would spread the dosage over the course of the day. Not all calcium supplements are created equal. Calcium citrate is better absorbed than calcium carbonate (found in Tums).

There may be reasons to "get milk" that go beyond calcium. Researchers in New Zealand have identified a protein present in both cows' milk and human breast milk that stimulates bone-forming cells in laboratory culture and that stimulates bone growth when injected into mice. The molecule, an iron-binding protein called lactoferrin, stimulates osteoblasts (bone-forming cells) and inhibits osteoclasts (cells that remove bone). Still experimental, lactoferrin holds promise for the prevention and treatment of osteoporosis. Also, one study showed that people who consume milk on a daily basis have a reduced risk of developing colorectal cancer. Vitamin D, in addition to calcium, was thought to be a factor in this protective effect.

Bone Density—Where Do You Stand?

The best way to measure bone density and determine if you have, or are getting, osteo-

ARE YOU AT RISK FOR OSTEOPOROSIS?

The following are considered risk factors for osteoporosis:

- **History of fracture as an adult**
- **Family history of fractures or osteoporosis**
- **Cigarette smoking**
- **Slight build or underweight**
- **White or Asian female**
- **Eating disorder**
- **Early menopause or hysterectomy**
- **Sedentary lifestyle**
- **Alcohol abuse**
- **Low-calcium diet**
- **Vitamin D deficiency, including inadequate sunlight exposure**
- **High caffeine intake**
- **Certain medical disorders (i.e., thyroid dysfunction) or the use of certain medications (Prednisone, corticosteroids, Dilantin)**

porosis is the DEXA (Dual Energy X-ray Absorptiometry) Scan. This is a safe, simple, and quick test using low-dose x-rays. The National Osteoporosis Foundation recommends a DEXA Scan for women over age 65 as well as younger women, or even men, considered at risk for osteoporosis. I often order a DEXA Scan for young, fit female athletes with recurrent stress fractures. Any woman who sustains a fracture, other than those with severe trauma involved, should be considered a candidate for a DEXA Scan. DEXA Scans can also be used to monitor bone gain or loss over time, and that is why a baseline test score is so important.

OTHER MINERALS

Our bodies require several key minerals, including potassium, chloride, sodium, magnesium, copper, zinc, and iron.

Potassium, chloride, and sodium are electrolytes, which means that they regulate the electrical potential of cell membranes. This makes them an essential element in conducting nerve impulses. To ensure normal functioning of our nerves and muscles, these three minerals have to be in proper balance.

Humans evolved on a diet rich in potassium (fruits and raw vegetables) and low in sodium. Our bodies responded to the challenge by finding ways to conserve sodium and excrete potassium, which in today's world, with today's typical diet of processed foods and not enough produce, is exactly the opposite of what's needed.

Sodium and chloride, combined, are what we ingest as salt, and our diet is awash in it. So an imbalance in this context usually means low potassium, which, even as a modest imbalance, can cause impaired blood-vessel tone, impaired muscle contraction, and, eventually, a loss of bone density. When you sweat a lot, part of what leaves your body is potassium.

The best source to replace this element comes in a convenient yellow package called a banana. Sports drinks market themselves as potassium replacements, but you'd have to drink 12 servings to obtain the potassium that's in one Chiquita. Other good sources of potassium are dark leafy green vegetables, tomatoes, cucumbers, zucchini, winter squash, carrots, turnips, onions, potatoes, apples, oranges, apricots, and strawberries.

Among other things, chloride helps carry carbon dioxide out of our cells and into our lungs. We need sodium after exercise to reduce the loss of liquids and to maintain the plasma osmolality that triggers our desire to drink. Pickles, pretzels, popcorn, and soy sauce are all good sources of sodium chloride (a.k.a. salt) when we're depleted.

Magnesium is a cofactor for many enzymes that support protein synthesis and thus wound repair, and most Americans don't get enough. This mineral gives structural stability to ATP, which supports collagen synthesis. It also protects against heart disease. Shoot for 400 milligrams daily, and the easiest way is to eat avocado, pumpkin seeds, and cashews.

Copper is necessary for development of connective tissue. It's also a powerful antioxidant, and it helps us metabolize iron. Whole wheat, honey, dried beans, and shellfish supply ample copper.

Zinc is a cofactor for RNA and DNA synthesis, protein synthesis, and cellular proliferation, which makes it a vitally important element for the repair or remodeling of your frame, especially after injury or surgery. You need 15 milligrams of zinc every day, and your best source is lean, red beef—the darker red the better. However, chicken, fish, and lentils are also excellent sources.

Lack of adequate iron is probably the most common nutritional deficiency in the world, especially among females, and among others maintaining a low body weight.

Iron supports collagen production, and you need 18 milligrams of iron every day. It may also protect against injury, at least among female athletes. One study of high school runners showed that, over the cross-country running season, the girls who sustained injuries averaged levels of ferritin, the body's primary iron-storage molecule, 40 percent lower than those who remained uninjured.

Iron is a key component of hemoglobin, which carries oxygen to muscle, so it may be that low ferritin, which suggests low oxygen delivery, leads to muscle fatigue, which then predisposes to injury. Low ferritin may also impede muscle and connective tissue repair, which means that small dinks can escalate into serious problems. Low blood-iron levels also reduce the oxidative potential in the muscles, which shifts over to metabolism that produces more lactate, which can cause muscle injuries.

VITAMINS

Vitamins are molecules that serve as catalysts, which means that they facilitate chemical reactions. If the catalysts are missing, normal body functions can break down and leave you weakened and more susceptible to disease and injury. Vitamin deficiency can even lead to DNA damage, the same way that exposure to x-rays can. This leads to premature aging and various degenerative diseases.

I recommend that you take a daily multivitamin supplement. I prefer Centrum to ensure a healthy frame. You need the following vitamins.

Vitamin A: An antioxidant important in wound healing, it helps maintain vision; promotes bone growth, cell differentiation, and healthy skin; and also helps to regulate the immune system.

The most usable form of A is retinol, which comes from liver and eggs. Some foods—dark green vegetables, fortified cereals—have beta-carotene, which converts to retinol, which is also an antioxidant and may lower your risk of cancer.

The best way to get the A you need is through five servings a day of dark green, leafy vegetables, and/or yellow or orange fruit and vegetables. This is especially true for vegetarians or vegans who don't eat eggs or dairy products.

B vitamins: Called the B-complex, these are actually a group of eight vitamins: thiamine (B_1), riboflavin (B_2), niacin (B_3), pyridoxine (B_6), folic acid (B_9), cyanocobalamin (B_{12}), pantothenic acid, and biotin. These serve as catalysts for the breakdown of carbohydrates into glucose for energy and the breakdown of fats and proteins to maintain the nervous system. They are also important in energy production at the cellular level.

The Bs play an indirect role in healing by boosting immunity. They also reduce levels of homocysteine, an amino acid implicated in heart attacks, strokes, and Alzheimer's, and now shown to be a culprit in osteoporosis as well. High homocysteine is associated with a twice as high rate of hip fractures.

All B vitamins are important, but the following serve special functions for your frame. Riboflavin (B_2) acts as a coenzyme for oxidation-reduction reactions throughout the body, which act to inhibit chemical reactions with oxygen or highly reactive free radicals that can cause cell damage. Vitamin B_{12} acts as a coenzyme in the synthesis and repair of DNA. B_{12} is also involved in producing red blood cells, protein synthesis, tissue repair, and maintaining bone health. Folic acid (B_9) is involved in protein synthesis and tissue repair, as well as helping to prevent hardening of the arteries. This we usually associate with cardiovascular disease, but you need healthy blood vessels not just for your heart and brain, but to bring nourishment to tendons, muscles, and ligaments as well. Deficiency in folic acid is one of the ways that your microcirculation can be compromised.

B vitamins are found in liver, whole-grain cereals, rice, nuts, milk, eggs, meats, fish, fruits, leafy green vegetables, and many other foods.

Vitamin C: Vitamin C, vital in forming collagen and in helping maintain capillaries, bones, and teeth, is one of your frame's most essential building blocks. It also helps in the absorption of iron, avoiding muscle soreness, and keeping up your immunity to colds. It is helpful in maintaining the health of your joints and may be important in the prevention and treatment of osteoarthritis. A study in the journal *Plastic and Reconstructive Surgery* found that an herbal "cocktail" containing vitamin C, bromelain (an anti-inflammatory enzyme found in pineapple), rutin (a flavenoid), and grapeseed extract accelerated wound healing and also noted that vitamin C can speed up healing of surgical wounds and some injuries.

The Daily Value for vitamin C for women is 75 milligrams, men 90, but I believe you need more for optimal frame function. Citrus fruits and tomatoes are the best sources, but C is added to many noncitrus juices and to fortified cereals. I recommend 1,000 milligrams of vitamin C daily and believe that my consistent use of vitamin C over the years is one of the biggest reasons that I have not missed a single day of work in well over 20 years!

Vitamin D: Also known as calciferol, vitamin D helps strengthen bones and stave off arthritis. The major biologic function of vitamin D is to maintain normal blood levels of calcium and phosphorus. Vitamin D aids in the absorption of calcium, helping to form and maintain strong bones. It promotes bone mineralization in concert with a number of other vitamins, minerals, and hormones. Without vitamin D, bones can become thin, brittle, soft, or misshapen, and low levels of D have been shown to be associated with low back pain.

Milk is most often fortified with 125 International Units (IU) of vitamin D per glass—one fourth of your minimum daily requirement. Breakfast cereals, pastries, breads, crackers, cereal grain bars, and other foods may be forti-fied with 10 to 15 percent of the Daily Value for vitamin D. There is also some vitamin D in eggs, organ meats, and fish such as salmon, sardines, and herring. But by and large there are no single foods rich in D, which is why supplementary D is a good idea for many people, especially seniors whose bodies no longer convert D to its active form quite as well.

Vitamin D is also manufactured in the skin after direct exposure to sunlight. The trouble is, people spend less time outdoors and (rightly) take precautions against sun exposure for fear of skin cancer. Also, places as far north as Boston receive virtually no UVB rays, the ultraviolet light that synthesizes D, between October and March. Sunscreens with a sun protection factor of 8 or greater will block UV rays that produce vitamin D, but it's still important to routinely use sunscreen whenever sun exposure is longer than 10 to 15 minutes. On the other hand, limited sun exposure increases the importance of good sources of vitamin D in your diet.

During menopause, more bone is being broken down (reabsorbed) than rebuilt. Estrogen replacement, which limits symptoms of menopause, can help slow down the development of osteoporosis by stimulating the activity of cells that rebuild bone. But concerns over the possible relation of estrogen replacement to the development of certain cancers prevents many women from relying on supplements.

Vitamin D deficiency has been associated with greater incidence of hip fractures in older people, especially women. Since bone loss increases the risk of fractures, vitamin D supplementation may help prevent fractures resulting from osteoporosis. Individuals who have a reduced ability to absorb dietary fat (fat malabsorption) may need extra vitamin D because it is a fat-soluble vitamin.

If you have been told to take a vitamin D supplement, a dose between 400 and 800 IU per day is safe and potent. Older patients should take the 800 IU/day dose. Almost all multivitamins contain 400 IU/day. Also, vitamin D supplements can be bought at most drugstores, food stores, and health food stores. Many calcium supplements also contain vitamin D in the right amount.

Vitamin E: An antioxidant, vitamin E maintains and stabilizes cell membranes against free radicals. E can also function as a sort of nontoxic steroid to reduce inflammation. Extra E has helped individuals with a variety of musculoskeletal conditions including rheumatoid arthritis, osteoarthritis, fibromyalgia, and lupus. It can be a painkiller, reduce cardiovascular risk, and also boost immune function. Recently, there has been some conflicting health data about vitamin E supplements. Your best bet is to get this vitamin naturally through food. Good sources include hazelnuts, sweet potatoes, and peanut butter.

Vitamin K: This is a fat-soluble vitamin that promotes clotting factors in the blood as well as general bone health. Low levels of K are associated with hip fractures. The best sources of K are green vegetables and soy.

ANTIOXIDANTS

We've already discussed the harm that can be created by "free radicals," the byproducts of oxidation that can throw a monkey wrench into the workings of your cells, especially those in your musculoskeletal system. To trump those wild cards, you need antioxidants, both for recovery from workouts and for preventing, or at least limiting, osteoarthritis, tendinopathy, and other bone and joint problems.

Even Ken Cooper, MD, the father of the aerobic movement (he coined the term "aerobics"), who I worked with on the President's Council on Physical Fitness and Sports and respect greatly, now believes that his years of running and high-power aerobic exercise has resulted in significant oxidative free radical damage. He now favors lower intensity workouts with less metabolic cost to your system, in combination with antioxidant and other vitamin supplementation.

When we exercise, the body uses oxygen to form ATP, which allows the muscles to contract. Unfortunately, the breakdown of oxygen is not 100 percent clean, and the waste product is free radicals such as superoxides, hyperoxides, and hydroxyls.

The more training you do, the more oxygen you use, and the more your body forms these free radicals. Their damage to the muscle cells triggers the inflammatory response we associate with muscle soreness after vigorous training. But the good news is that antioxidants in the diet—led by vitamins C and E (tocopherol)—can help prevent this kind of injury. And once again, proper exercise plays its medicinal role. A Harvard Medical School study has shown that exercise combined with vitamin E reduced free radicals far better than either vitamin E or exercise alone.

This means that athletes in regular training who modestly supplement their diets with C and E not only reduce their injury risks, but they can also train harder without as much soreness.

Other free radical fighters are the 4,000 natural bioflavonoid compounds, including the flavones, flavonols, and isoflavones found in many common foods.

For your frame, one of the most important of these is the proanthocyanidins (PCOs), which are free-radical scavengers that also inhibit the activity of enzymes that can break down key protein structures within tendons, ligaments, and cartilage during inflammation. In addition, they facilitate an enzyme called proline hydroxylase, that is absolutely essential for the synthesis of collagen.

Foods rich in PCOs include cabbage, rhubarb, blueberries, currants, cranberries, grapes, raspberries, strawberries, and red wine, one glass of which contains 150 milligrams of PCOs.

Quercetin, another bioflavonoid, also seems to have pronounced anti-inflammatory properties. In one study, quercetin was able to reduce the production of free radicals by 33 percent, and the release of protein-degrading enzymes by 52 percent. Other research suggested that quercetin tends to dampen the release of histamine, the chemical that helps produce the airway-tightening effect associated with exercise-induced asthma. Foods high in quercetin include parsley, sage, onions, kale, red wine, broccoli, French beans, and apples.

Happily, many other great sources of the antioxidants you need are very tasty and easy to work into your diet, chief among them blueberries, tomatoes, and strawberries. But to really get it right, you need to cover the whole spectrum of colors—pigment power, they call it—because different fruits and vegetables have different nutrients. Some pack more punch through their higher natural concentrations of micronutrients. So the idea is to eat a rainbow.

Red: The aforementioned tomatoes (but especially cooked tomatoes), as well as pink grapefruit and watermelon. These contain carotenoid lycopene, an antioxidant known to protect against prostate cancer, lung cancer, and heart disease.

Darker red to purple: In addition to blueber-

■ ■ ■ BEST FOODS FOR ANTIOXIDANTS

Nutrition scientists at the U.S. Department of Agriculture (USDA) used the latest technologies available to identify the foods that contain the most antioxidants per serving.

Here they are, ranked from most antioxidants per serving to least:

1. Small red beans (dried)
2. Wild blueberries
3. Red kidney beans
4. Pinto beans
5. Blueberries (cultivated)
6. Cranberries
7. Artichokes (cooked)
8. Blackberries
9. Prunes
10. Raspberries
11. Strawberries
12. Red Delicious apples
13. Granny Smith apples
14. Pecans
15. Sweet cherries
16. Black plums
17. Russet potatoes (cooked)
18. Black beans (dried)
19. Plums
20. Gala apples

ries and strawberries, eat plums, red apples (be sure to eat the skin), beets, eggplant, red cabbage, and red peppers. These provide anthocyanins, which help prevent blood clots.

Reddish orange: Carrots, mangoes, cantaloupe, winter squash, and sweet potatoes have beta-carotene that protects the skin against free radical damage and promotes repair of DNA.

Yellow/orange: That fruit from Florida, along with peaches, papaya, and nectarines, have beta crytothanxin, which helps cellular communication and fights heart disease.

Yellow/green: Spinach, corn, green peas, avocado, and honeydew melon contain lutein and zeaxanthin, which reduce the risk of cataracts and age-related macular degeneration, a cause of blindness.

Green: Broccoli, brussels sprouts, cabbage, kale, and bok choy. These contain sulforaphane, isocyanate, and indoles, which help to fight cancer.

White/green: Garlic, onions, leeks, celery, asparagus, pears, and green grapes, including those used in white wine. These contain allicin, which fights tumors and antioxidant flavonoids such as quercetin and kaempferol.

In addition, I recommend a daily antioxidant supplement including 1,000 milligrams of vitamin C. Also, Andrew Lessman's Ultimate Antioxidants (www.yourvitamins.com) is a great choice that combines 24 ingredients from berries, spices, tea, and other natural sources.

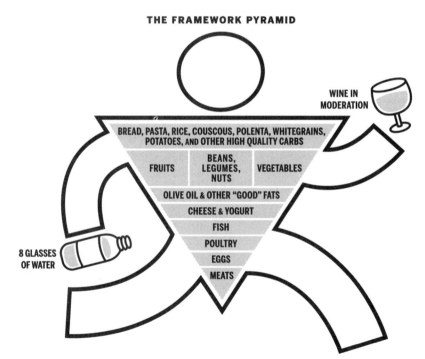

THE FRAMEWORK PYRAMID

WINE IN MODERATION

BREAD, PASTA, RICE, COUSCOUS, POLENTA, WHITEGRAINS, POTATOES, AND OTHER HIGH QUALITY CARBS

FRUITS | BEANS, LEGUMES, NUTS | VEGETABLES

OLIVE OIL & OTHER "GOOD" FATS

CHEESE & YOGURT

FISH

POULTRY

EGGS

MEATS

8 GLASSES OF WATER

THE FRAMEWORK PYRAMIND STRESSES THE IMPORTANCE OF EXERCISE, NUTRITION, AND THE ROLE OF THE MIND IN CREATING AND MAINTAINING HEALTH. IT'S WHAT YOU EAT, WHAT EATS YOU, AND WHAT YOU DO (OR DON'T DO) REGULARLY THAT MAKES THE DIFFERENCE.

LA DOLCE VITA

After all this analysis, happily, the easiest way to stay with this athlete's diet is to enjoy yourself with great Mediterranean cuisine! If you've ever been to southern France, Italy, Greece, or Spain, you know that life there revolves around plenty of sunshine, wine, grapes, grains, fish, olives, and tomatoes. In other words, eating smart can be a great source of pleasure.

It's not for nothing that the incidence of coronary disease on the island of Crete is 37 times lower than in the United States. The *New England Journal of Medicine* estimates that the Mediterranean diet can lower your overall risk of mortality by 25 percent. (They also found that 1 hour of vigorous exercise daily reduced the risk of mortality by 28 percent!)

This Mediterranean diet is ideal for your frame. It is high in protein, but it does not scrimp on the grains and other carbohydrates you need for energy to sustain a workout. But this diet recommends complex carbohydrates, like whole wheat and brown rice rather than refined carbohydrates.

Twenty-five to 35 percent of the calories in a Mediterranean diet come from good fats like olive oil, which is high in phenolic antioxidants; 50 percent come from complex carbohydrates that require your body to work harder to break down the sugars. This takes time and provides better insulin regulation and sustained release for your workout. Plus, the extra fiber is much better for your digestion and the health of your colon. It is also rich in antioxidants and phytonutrients, as well as alpha-linolenic acid, which converts to the omega-3 fatty acids that are good for your heart and joints. Mediterranean diets also have been shown to be anti-inflammatory, reducing systemic markers of inflammation, something important not only for heart health but also for your joints and tendons.

Despite a relatively high fat percentage, only 7 or 8 percent of the calories are from the bad saturated fats—far less than consumed by most U.S. dieters. It's the good things in olive oil, combined with other antioxidants in wine, fruit, and vegetables, that work together to lower the risk of heart disease and cancer and at the same time protect your frame.

In addition to tasting great, the athlete's/Mediterranean diet feeds your frame by strengthening, fortifying, lubricating, repairing, regenerating, putting out the fires of unwanted inflammation, and taking out the trash of free radical damage.

THE RIGHT WEIGHT FOR YOU

In addition to all the other reasons to stay at your ideal weight—cardiovascular health, looking good, and feeling good, plus being able to move the way you want to—avoiding excess pounds is better for your frame. For every extra pound you carry, your hips and knees feel the effect of 5 extra pounds. If you're 10 pounds overweight, that means 50 extra pounds for your knees to carry around.

This is why excess weight is a major risk factor for osteoarthritis, and why losing even a little weight can help. Being overweight also results in more rapid progression of arthritis once it is present. Those extra pounds are also a factor in low back conditions such as disk degeneration and disk herniation. Less weight to carry means less stress and strain on those bones and joints.

However, some athletes, especially distance runners, and even more especially female distance runners, border on a level of skinniness that is not good for their health or for their athletic performance. They can develop the "Female Athlete Triad" consisting of disordered eating, amenorrhea (the cessation of their monthly periods), and osteoporosis. Once again, we have to acknowledge the "dose response" of exercise, which is to say that "more" is not always better.

The minimal level of body fat for good health is 5 percent for males and 12 percent for females. However, the danger of having too little body fat is not foremost on the minds of most Americans.

Sixty-five percent of us are either obese or overweight. Thirty percent of us are obese, and 35 percent could lose some weight.

No surprise—Americans spend far more time driving cars and watching TV than they do exercising. We also work longer hours than anyone else in the developed world, which not only cuts into our time for physical activities, it messes up our eating habits. We now spend half our food dollars eating out, where the emphasis seems to be on quantity rather than quality.

In fact, one quarter of the calories consumed by Americans come from junk food, with soft drinks accounting for 7.1 percent of the total! These "foods" are essentially empty calories, with no nutritional value, and that's before you add in all the harmful effects. Our foods are overly processed, sugary, starchy, greasy, salty, and trans-fat rich.

But it's not just that we eat badly; we simply eat too much. The Centers for Disease Control and Prevention found that, in 2000, women consumed 22 percent more calories a day than they did in 1971! Men in 2000 consumed 8 percent more, but that may mean that they were already overeating in 1971.

We've become "super-sized" people because, for a generation, we've been "super sizing" our portions. The first McDonald's burgers were 1.6 ounces; the Big Mac and Quarter Pounder are now 4 ounces. In 1916, a bottle of Coke was 6.5 ounces. Now the standard size is 12 ounces, with the 20-ounce chugalug coming on strong. Pricing down at the convenience store makes this shift almost inevitable—people see that big plastic bottle as a better value proposition, when what they should see is that much more sugar and empty calories.

A nutritionist at New York University tells us that, compared with 1971, the recipes used in cookbooks and newspapers call for the same amount of ingredients, but the number of servings they say the recipe will yield has shrunk. In other words, we assume that everyone will eat more.

Keeping your weight where you want it isn't rocket science, or something that requires Jennifer Garner's personal trainer. The essential long-term factor is simply output versus intake. Eat less, move more.

Your body mass index (BMI) gives you a rough idea of your ideal weight. For adults, normal BMI is below 25. Those with BMI between 25 and 29.9 are considered overweight, between 30 and 39.9 obese, and those over 40 are characterized with extreme obesity. BMI can sometimes be deceptive, though. Two people can have the same BMI,

BODY MASS INDEX (BMI)

HEIGHT   WEIGHT (IN POUNDS)

HEIGHT																				
4'10"	91	96	100	105	110	115	119	124	129	134	138	143	148	153	158	162	167	172	177	181
4'11"	94	99	104	109	114	119	124	128	133	138	143	148	153	158	163	168	173	178	183	188
5'0"	97	102	107	112	118	123	128	133	138	143	148	153	158	163	168	174	179	184	189	194
5'1"	100	106	111	116	122	127	132	137	143	148	153	158	164	169	174	180	185	190	195	201
5'2"	104	109	115	120	126	131	136	142	147	153	158	164	169	175	180	186	191	196	202	207
5'3"	107	113	118	124	130	135	141	146	152	158	163	169	175	180	186	191	197	203	208	214
5'4"	110	116	122	128	134	140	145	151	157	163	169	174	180	186	192	197	204	209	215	221
5'5"	114	120	126	132	138	144	150	156	162	168	174	180	186	192	198	204	210	216	222	228
5'6"	118	124	130	136	142	148	155	161	167	173	179	186	192	198	204	210	216	223	229	235
5'7"	121	127	134	140	146	153	159	166	172	178	185	191	198	204	211	217	223	230	236	242
5'8"	125	131	138	144	151	158	164	171	177	184	190	197	203	210	216	223	230	236	243	249
5'9"	128	135	142	149	155	162	169	176	182	189	196	203	209	216	223	230	236	248	250	257
5'10"	132	139	146	153	160	167	174	181	188	195	202	209	216	222	229	236	243	250	257	264
5'11"	136	143	150	157	165	172	179	186	193	200	208	215	222	229	236	243	250	257	265	272
6'0"	140	147	154	162	169	177	184	191	199	206	213	221	228	235	242	250	258	265	272	279
6'1"	144	151	159	166	174	182	189	197	204	212	219	227	235	242	250	257	265	272	280	288
6'2"	148	155	163	171	179	186	194	202	210	218	225	233	241	249	256	264	272	280	287	295
6'3"	152	160	168	176	184	192	200	208	216	224	232	240	248	256	264	272	279	287	295	303
6'4"	156	164	172	180	189	197	205	213	221	230	238	246	254	263	271	279	287	295	304	312
	19	20	21	22	23	24	25	26	27	28	29	30	31	32	33	34	35	36	37	38

but a different percent body fat. (Think of the bodybuilder who carries 30 extra pounds of muscle versus the couch potato who carries 30 extra pounds of flab.)

The more meaningful measure is the tightness of your waistband, or the tone in those hips and thighs. Can you "pinch an inch"? And how do you look in the mirror in your birthday suit?

Keep in mind, too, that not everyone is meant to look like a Hollywood starlet or her lean, mean leading man. Some bodies were simply designed to carry a little more gravitas, so you have to be realistic—which also suggests a certain amount of self-acceptance.

Each person's metabolism and body type has a "set point" that acts like a thermometer. If you diet to slim down below your natural set point, your body will fight you all the way to return to the weight that your genes say is more natural for you.

Storing up even more fat is nature's response to lean times, even when the lean times occur by choice, which explains why crash diets don't work in the long term. Making matters worse, when faced with sudden caloric restriction, your body is programmed to burn muscle as fuel before it ever draws down into its stores of deep fat, which it guards as precious fuel for emergencies only.

Severe diet restrictions also make metabolic rates drop by as much as half, which defeats your purpose. The early drop in scale weight you might see from a fad diet is usually a combination of water loss and muscle loss. Otherwise, you've played into the body's worst fear—starvation—which causes it to burn less fat and store more.

There are 3,500 calories in a pound, and most of us need a minimum of 1,200 calories a day just to keep things running at all.

If your normal diet is 2,000 calories a day and you weigh 200 pounds, you can lose a pound of stored fat in 7 days by lowering your intake to 1,500 calories a day (500 less a day × 7 days = 3,500 calories).

Exercise is vital, but, truth be told, you may burn only 8 to 10 calories a minute during a serious workout. At that rate, an hour on a treadmill may burn off 60 calories, which isn't really that much. That's why it's important not just to count calories, but to make every calorie count! If you're going to eat it, make sure it's worth it in terms of nutrition.

Keep in mind, too, that rapid weight loss will also sacrifice muscle. In fact, your body is programmed by millions of years of evolution to burn muscle as fuel before it draws down into its stores of deep fat, which are for emergencies only.

That's why strength training is so important, even when your primary objective is weight loss. Not only does it keep more calorie-burning muscle on your frame, but slowly, over time, it is possible to reset your set point, and that's where the benefit of exercise really kicks in.

Lean muscle burns more calories than other tissues, even when you're sleeping. Building up your muscle cells is also building a bigger calorie-burning furnace that burns day and night. Strength training also prevents the loss of muscle tissue that's otherwise sacrificed when your body senses that it is being "starved."

Watch your waistline, not the scale, because you may shed ugly fat and still find your weight staying the same or even going up a tad as you add healthful muscle.

And the great thing about those muscle cells is that their fires burn day and night, whether you're running 3 miles or getting a good night's sleep.

After the age of 30 or 40, we all naturally lose muscle as we age, which, again, lowers the metabolic rate. So, unless you counteract that natural decline through strength training, you'll put on weight simply by eating the same as you always have.

WEIGHT CONTROL FOR ACTIVE PEOPLE

All the relevant science tells us that weight control is determined by Q3—quantity, quality, and quotidian (time of day). What counts is how much you eat, the quality of the nutrients included, and the time of day in which you eat it. Calories consumed later in the day seem to have an easier time converting into fat. By contrast, high-quality calories consumed early in the day, as in a high-protein breakfast, will sustain you and decrease your hunger later.

But patience and perseverance are also factors.

Rather than starve yourself, you have to set your goal as lowering your weight over time and remember the only consistently successful long-term weight control programs include a combination of exercise and proper nutrition with calorie control. Either effort by itself, dieting or life on the stairclimber, will fail most of the time. While popular diets may get you motivated to lose those extra pounds and even give you a jumpstart, they probably won't sustain you. That's because most fad diets deprive you of necessary nutrients. Most people will regain lost weight, and more. The trick to sensible nutrition is to not cut yourself off from the pleasure of eating, which will only tighten the spring for a really disastrous rebound into gluttony as soon as your willpower hits a weak spot. Just change what you eat, and eat it in sensible portions—and get more exercise! You don't have to be as skinny as Gwyneth Paltrow to say that if you can't flex it, lose it!

SUPPLEMENTS

Your body absorbs nutrients much more readily from food than from a pill, so taking in the nutrients you need through what you eat is far more effective. However, for a variety of reasons, most of us do not get the full array of vitamins and other necessary micronutrients, and this is why I recommend the routine use of certain high-quality supplements in addition to "proper eating."

There are some 29,000 supplements available in the United States today, and they're regulated like food, not drugs, which means the government considers them safe unless proved otherwise. In practice, what this means is that no one is really watching what's in supplements and much more leeway is given in terms of false claims and blatantly false advertising.

Without FDA regulation, you have no certainty of what you're getting. And study after study has shown that what you get is often not what's advertised.

In 2001, in fact, an Olympic committee found that 15 percent of supplements had steroid precursors that weren't listed. Banned substances such as androstenedione and ephedrine show up all the time. Impurities can find their way into the product. Some nutrients, taken to excess, can do damage, and some supplements may interact with prescription drugs. A study of the top 10 brands of the joint supplement glucosamine and chondroitin sulfate showed that only two or three brands actually contained what they claimed on the label. Most brands have much less than claimed and a few, in beautiful packages, had absolutely no active ingredient! Another study revealed that 84 percent of brands did not meet label claims in terms of ingredients.

Reputable manufacturers have banded together in a voluntary organization to test for purity, potency, and uniformity, and to assign the United States Pharmacopeia (USP) seal of approval for products that can prove that they are everything they say they are.

So let the buyer beware. Just because you found it in a health food store doesn't mean it's healthful or even safe.

One supplement I can recommend whole-heartedly is the double-strength Cosamin® DS brand of glucosamine and chondroitin sulfate, because here the positive effects have been scientifically proven. This combination has been shown to be effective in reducing joint symptoms, possibly by promoting cartilage production and repair. The usual starting dosage includes 1,500 milligrams of glucosamine and 1,200 milligrams of chondroitin sulfate in divided doses.

Cosamin® DS includes not only glucosamine and chondroitin sulfate but also manganese and ascorbate (vitamin C). Glucosamine contains a key component of the matrix of connective tissue, especially articular cartilage. Cosamin® DS also has the only low molecular weight chondroitin sulfate in the United States and this higher quality, lower molecular weight version is absorbed more efficiently. Chondroitin sulfate also inhibits enzymes that degrade or damage articular cartilage, and it increases the production of hyaluronic acid, a natural joint lubricant.

Glucosamine and chondroitin sulfate are considered very safe and also numerous scientific studies have shown them to be effective in the treatment of osteoarthritis. I recommend Cosamin® DS to all my patients with osteoarthritis as well as many recovering from certain types of knee injuries or surgery including many of the pro basketball players, dancers, and other athletes who are under my care. There is some research data that suggests that glucosamine and chondroitin sulfate may prevent the progression of osteoarthritis, but the jury is still out.

These supplements do not help everyone, and the benefits can come slowly, sometimes taking 2 to 3 months to kick in. So my advice is to try it for a 2-month minimum before deciding whether you are responsive.

Studies suggest that glucosamine may also enhance the power of ibuprofen (i.e., Motrin or Advil) to relieve pain and thus may allow lower dosing of ibuprofen in treating a variety of bone and joint problems. And even these familiar painkillers require a note of caution. NSAIDs can be helpful to your joints in general, but they can also have negative consequences for your frame. There is evidence that they can slow fracture healing and block your body's internal mechanisms for repairing damage to your joint surfaces. This may even be true of ligaments and tendon healing as well. Many people have other problems with NSAIDs, including stomach ulcers, gastric bleeding, and renal troubles so don't go popping any of these pills in your mouth like candy.

Side effects are one of the reasons that, for inflammation and other joint issues, I recommend careful use of NSAIDs in the short run, unless otherwise prescribed by your doctor, and for the long haul, chondroitin sulfate and glucosamine.

Other supplements that are worth considering include the following.

PCO: This antioxidant, available in certain foods, is also commercially available in supplements known as pine-bark extract, pycnogenol or grapeseed extract.

PCO protects against oxidative stress and

acts as a free radical scavenger. Pycnogenol also dilates small blood vessels leading to muscle tissues.

In one study, 10 healthy volunteers, over a 30-day period, took a daily dose of 110 milligrams of PCO extracted from grapes. The levels of vitamin E in red-blood-cell membranes increased by 56 percent, concentrations of degraded DNA in blood plasma dropped (degraded DNA is a sign of oxidant damage), and there was a shift to a higher level of polyunsaturated fatty acids in red-cell membranes. Another study showed that grapeseed extract could neutralize free radicals 50 times better than vitamins E or C.

ASU: There is an interesting product derived from avocado and soybean oils called Piascledin, available in France by prescription. There it has been studied for 15 years, and it appears to increase production of chondrocytes, the cartilage-producing cells in your joints, and thus helps ease the effects of osteoarthritis.

In the meantime, you can get the same substance at healthfood stores under the name Avocado-Soybean Unsaponifiable, or ASU. Nutramax Labs has a high quality brand Avoca that combines ASU with glucosamine.

Limbrel (flavocoxid): A safe, natural "medical food" (i.e., requires a prescription), Limbrel is thought to both reduce pain and prevent cartilage loss in osteoarthritis through its anti-inflammatory and antioxidant properties. Learn more at www.Limbrel.com.

SAM-e: SAM-e (S-Adenosyl-methionine) is an over-the-counter dietary supplement used to treat osteoarthritis. It is synthesized in the body from the essential amino acid methionine. Some studies have shown effectiveness in reducing joint symptoms but more research is needed before this can be definitively recommended.

OTHER RESOURCES FOR ACHY BONES AND JOINTS

Zyflamend is a combination of ginger, turmeric, and other anti-inflammatory agents. High doses can cause a burning sensation in the stomach, so always take it with food.

Boswellian is an herb from Ayurvedic medicine, available in capsules, that reduces inflammation and improves blood supply to the joints.

Ginger is a natural anti-inflammatory that can be taken in pills in daily amounts from 500 to 1,000 milligrams. You have to give it time to show any effect, because it takes a while to build up.

Turmeric, the antioxidant in yellow mustard, is available as an extract in 400 to 600 milligram dosages, but it, too, has to build up for 8 weeks or so before it will reduce inflammation.

L-arginine is an amino acid that may stimulate insulin production (insulin is one of the body's most potent tissue-building hormones), enhance the production of critical protein structures, improve immune function, and also increase the synthesis of nitric and nitrous oxide, which dilate blood vessels and promote the delivery of oxygen to damaged tissues.

Cayenne pepper contains capsaicin, which triggers the body to release endorphins, natural opiates.

Willow bark contains salicin, a natural anti-inflammatory substance and precursor to acetylsalicylic acid (aspirin)

Acetyl-L-carnitine, plus alpha lipoic acid, is an "anti-aging" compound being marketed over the Internet by a company called Juvenon. There has been at least one credible study showing older mice "getting up and doing the Macarena" when given the substance, and it is now undergoing clinical trials. Supposedly it works by protecting the mitochondria, the "furnaces" where oxygen is burning to create energy.

Gamma linolenic acid (GLA) assists omega-3 fats to make beneficial, anti-inflammatory prostaglandins. Good sources of GLA include evening primrose, black currant seed, and borage seed oils, but it's also available in capsules.

Branched-chain amino acids may be beneficial for recovery from injury. Glutamine has been linked with improved connective-tissue repair, ornithine is believed to stimulate wound healing, and phenylalanine may reduce the pain associated with musculoskeletal trauma.

Coenzyme Q10 may neutralize free radicals within the mitochondria, preserving mitochondrial integrity. Likewise carotenoids, zinc, and niacinamide.

THE ULTIMATE NO-NO

This may seem painfully obvious to anyone reading a fitness book, but just about the worst thing you can do for your frame is to abuse alcohol or smoke.

Alcoholism is a major contributor to osteoporosis. And in North America, the primary category of adults with vitamin deficiencies are alcoholics.

Thiamine deficiency is common in heavy drinkers, because alcohol interferes with the absorption of thiamine through the intestines. People who drink too much often are deficient in vitamins A, B_6, and B_{12}. Excess alcohol intake also depletes your stores of A, but vitamin A supplements may increase liver toxicity.

So the nutritional solution is pretty obvious—two glasses of wine a day, tops. If you have trouble sticking to that, or if you have had prior alcohol-related problems, it might be time to consider a more serious intervention, especially if you have a family history of alcoholism.

My equally obvious—and equally urgent—recommendation is to not smoke and to stay away from those who do.

When I was a surgical resident, it was just then becoming possible for hand specialists to reattach severed fingers. Smoking was still allowed in hospitals in those days, and we used to see recovering patients take a puff on a cigarette, only to have their newly reattached finger turn blue! That's how badly nicotine restricts blood flow to the small vessels. Just as your heart depends on your coronary arteries, your muscles, tendons, and bones rely on small networks of blood vessels for their ongoing nourishment and rejuvenation. Even secondhand smoke from a friend smoking in the room, or even down the hall, was enough to cut off the circulation and lower the oxygen levels in those fingers.

Smoking is a risk factor for osteoporosis.

Also, bones, like wounds, just don't heal as well with nicotine in the system, and infection rates are higher. That's why some surgeons refuse to do spinal fusions on smokers. We don't yet have definitive evidence, but I strongly suspect that tendon problems are also exacerbated by smoking. It has been shown to wrinkle your collagen-rich skin, especially on your face through microcirculation damage, and I believe it does the same to collagen throughout your frame, especially your tendons. Smoking also interferes with the microcirculation in the disks (shock absorbers) in your spine, and smokers have higher incidents of back pain, as well as degenerating and herniated disks. Smokers who undergo general and orthopedic surgery have a higher incidence of wound infections than nonsmokers. Healing problems go even deeper. Fractures, too, will heal more slowly in smokers and in some instances actually not heal at all, something we call a nonunion, which are definitely more common in those who inhale.

NUTRITION AND YOUR FRAME: THE BOTTOM LINE

If you want to look like an athlete, perform like an athlete, and bounce back like an athlete, then you should eat like an athlete—not a teenage one-hit wonder, but a proven athlete with staying power.

Strive for a nutritious diet composed of 50 to 60 percent carbs, 12 to 20 percent protein, and no more than 30 percent fats. Remember both quantity and quality count. Strive for complex carbs, not refined sugary ones. Learn more about reading food labels (you are indeed what you eat) as well as the glycemic index, especially as it relates to pre- and post-workout fuel. The right kinds of fats are good for you but watch out, the calories can add up quickly. The more intense your workouts, the greater your protein needs. Meat packs a punch, but there are also great vegetarian sources.

Your body needs many micronutrients, and they usually can best be gotten through wise food choices. However, it does not hurt to supplement with a multivitamin and antioxidant supplement to assure you get what you need. Calcium and vitamin D, too, are important, especially for women, starting in their teens.

If you have bone and joint issues, then it is even more important that you get the full array of necessary micronutrients as well as additional supplements covered in this section. Brand does matter, so buyer beware.

If you want to lose or gain weight, learn to count calories and manage them like you would a bank account. 3,500 calories equals one pound. If you consume 300 extra calories a day (i.e., one big soda), you will gain a pound in about 2 weeks! It adds up quickly. It also works the other way. Simple measures, like reducing the lower quality calories in your diet, result in sustainable weight loss, especially when combined with exercise. Always gravitate toward high-quality food choices and avoid the naked calories.

Also, water, water everywhere. Your cells are not much different than that of your houseplant, and you know what that looks like when you forget to water it. Proper nutrition and hydration make for powerful frame fuel and thus an essential step in the FrameWork plan. A few years ago Governor Schwarzenegger introduced me to Jack La Lanne, the grand old man of fitness. Jack is a living legend and an inspiration for all. The man opened the first modern American health club in 1936. In 1951, he became the first fitness guru on TV, with a show that lasted until 1985. Ninety years old as of this writing, Jack is still going strong, a testament to being built to last. Two of his famous phrases have stayed with me. One of these is that "your waistline is your lifeline." The other brings it all together: "Exercise is king. Nutrition is queen. Put them together, and you've got a kingdom."

40 FOODS TO FORTIFY YOUR FRAME

As I've tried to make clear, eating right isn't just about staying thin and feeding your frame properly doesn't have to be a hardship assignment. To drive home the point, here are 40 foods—quick and easy—that can help ensure that you're built to last.

1. Chocolate! A study at Cornell University in Ithaca, New York, has shown that hot cocoa has twice the antioxidants as red wine. But take it easy (watching the calories) and take it straight. Go for the simple squares of dark chocolate, not milk chocolate, and avoid the creamy nougat and coconut filling.

2. Blueberries and strawberries. These are two of the foods highest in antioxidants. Rinse them off, and they're ready to eat. Put them on cereal or simply pop them in your mouth.

3. Almonds and walnuts. These are a great source of vitamin E—1 ounce contains 8 milligrams. Almonds also contain unsaturated fats that reduce inflammation and help lubricate your tissues. A great source of omega-3 fatty acids including alpha-linoleic acid, walnuts are thought to inhibit production of neurotransmitters such as substance P and bradykinins, which increase pain and inflammation.

4. Sunflower seeds. A quarter cup contains 7 milligrams of vitamin E.

5. Pineapple. High in bromelain, pineapple is a natural anti-inflamatory agent and is especially helpful in reducing swelling, bruising, and pain in musculoskeletal injuries, as well as arthritis, bursitis, tendonitis, and carpal tunnel syndrome.

6. Honey. It contains antioxidants called phenolics. The darker the honey, the better.

7. Ginger. This is a natural anti-inflammatory agent.

8. Green tea (any tea, actually). The *Archives of Internal Medicine* in 2002 reported that drinking tea over the long term contributes to denser bones at the three sites measured, including the lower back. Tea contains fluoride, phytoestrogens, and a group of antioxidants known as flavonoids that we think work together to increase bone density. (Green tea also contains L-theanine, an amino acid that is antianxiety, so it has a calming effect.)

9. Mustard. Unlike its fattier cousin mayonnaise, this condiment—or at least the bright yellow American version—contains turmeric, which is an anti-inflammatory. It also stimulates circulation. Mustard greens contain loads of calcium, phosphorus, magnesium, and B vitamins.

10. Soy. This bean, which feeds most of the planet, contains isoflavone, a phyto-estrogen that the body readily accepts. It's an antioxidant that speeds muscle recovery after exercise, reducing soreness and inflammation. Studies show that, for girls, high levels of soy consumed in the teen years leads to reduced breast cancer later, less osteoporosis, and, well down the road, less severe symptoms of menopause. In another study, a supplement derived from tofu gave a 3.6 percent increase in bone density to postmenopausal women. Tofu actually tastes great in a stir-fry or on a salad.

11. Oatmeal. It's the real breakfast of champions. For years, Quaker Oats and Cheerios have touted the fact that oats can lower your cholesterol. But the rest of the story is that, as a complex carbohydrate, oatmeal has the added benefit of a slow release of energy rather than a spike and a plunge. But the less refined the oats (sorry, Cheerios) the better. Also, stove cooked oatmeal is a better choice, when time allows, than instant or microwave.

12. Dark bread with a lot of fiber. (The whiter the bread, the sooner you're dead!) Most American breads are like eating cotton candy, even the ones that call themselves "whole wheat." If you can squeeze the package too easily, keep trying until you find a much coarser bread.

13. Quinoa. A great alternative to rice, this grain (actually, it's the seed of a plant similar to spinach) is a complete protein with more vitamins and minerals than just about anything. Eaten for centuries in Peru, it's now making its way into American supermarkets.

14. Buckwheat. Likewise, not a true grain, this herb from Asia is incredibly nutritious. If you like pancakes now and then, it's really not that hard to make them from scratch using Egg Beaters, if you like, and throw in some buckwheat. (Then do a little extra workout to make use of all those carbs.)

15. Shrimp and crab. These foods have picked up a bad rap because of their high-cholesterol content, but their cholesterol is a kind that isn't easily absorbed into the body. They contain high protein with lots of minerals, and they're very easy to fix.

16. Salmon. High in omega-3 fatty acids, this fish is now farm-raised, relatively inexpensive, and hard not to trip over in restaurants and supermarkets. And that's a good thing, because it gives you healthy cell membranes, improves your joint functioning, and lowers your risk of heart disease. Spritz it with some lemon, throw it on the grill or under the broiler in your stove, and cook it 5 minutes per side. What could be easier? This is a gourmet dish you can make in 10 minutes that will taste just as good at home as it would in the fanciest restaurant. And leftovers? Toss them in a salad, cold, and you're ready to go.

17. Sardines. The taste is a little strong for some, but they are loaded with omega-3, and they come in a can! Open and eat. Anchovies? Same thing. And if you occasionally want something to go underneath your furry fish. . .

18. Pizza. If you stick to the thin crusts and go easy on the cheese, pizza can be just fine. The cooked tomatoes are actually a great source of lycopene, which can reduce your cancer risk, especially prostate. You have olive oil for the omega-3s, and if you pick your toppings carefully—red, green, and yellow peppers; olives; onions; mushrooms—you can eat your vitamin and mineral-enriched, antioxidant rainbow and have your pizza, too.

19. Tuna. This "chicken of the sea" is high in omega-3, but because these big fish are at the top of the food chain, you have to worry about their mercury content. Farm-raised salmon is the safer way to go, with tuna as an occasional treat.

20. Bananas. As previously mentioned, these guys come in a convenient, easy open package, and they're loaded with potassium to help regulate muscle metabolism and restore losses from exercise.

21. Oranges. The C in citrus will help with muscle soreness and help keep away colds by boosting your immunity. Want one that fits in your pocket? Try a clementine.

22. Cantaloupe. Aside from vitamins A and C and beta-carotene, this melon has the great advantages of tasting great and filling you

up. If you've ever had prosciutto y melon in an Italian restaurant, you know how great it can taste. Guess what? You can get prosciutto in just about any decent grocery store—it's expensive, but you don't need much. Slice a melon, lay some of that delicate, thinly sliced ham on top, and you are in culinary heaven.

23. Beans. Pinto, lentil, garbanzo, split pea—these are filled with protein and iron. Homemade split pea soup with chunks of ham or pancetta is another very easy meal that's filling and healthful to boot.

24. Carrots. These guys are filled with vitamin A and fiber, but how do you get yourself eating more of them? Carrot soup is one way. Or, much simpler, keep a bag of baby carrots front and center when you open your refrigerator.

25. Celery. Munch it straight or dip the stalks in natural peanut butter. And don't let it wilt in the crisper—make celery soup! It's easy—some chopped celery and onions in canned chicken broth or chicken bouillon. It takes 15 minutes, and you can freeze the leftovers.

26. Broccoli. High in potassium and antioxidants, this stuff is fantastic when lightly steamed. Look for the nearly bite-sized broccoli florets at your grocers. You can munch them cold and crisp.

27. Asparagus. Again, rich in vitamins A and C, steam it lightly for a great warm side dish, then keep the leftovers handy in the fridge. Cold asparagus is great to munch on, throw on a salad, or fold into an omelette.

28. Lettuce. Lots of vitamins A and C, but the darker the lettuce the better. My favorite is romaine, which has a satisfying crunch. In the last few years, restaurants have taken the salad to new heights, so observe and imitate. Salad doesn't have to be boring. Throw in some sunflower seeds, some tofu, a little olive oil, and balsamic vinegar, and you're golden. Walnuts, grapes, slices of pear, chunks of feta or blue cheese, anchovies, and olives—with a twist of lemon . . . make your own rules. And don't forget your colors—add the radicchio and the yellow peppers.

29. Spinach. Maybe Popeye was so strong because of his favorite vegetable's high content of vitamin E and alpha-linolenic acid, an omega-3 fatty acid and anti-inflammatory compound. It's also high in B–complex vitamins. Try it the Italian way—throw a little chopped garlic in the pan, some olive oil, steam the freshly washed spinach, then spritz it with lemon. It's great in salads, too, and even richer in nutrients than lettuce. Try fresh spinach, mandarin oranges, and pine nuts, with just a little olive oil as dressing.

30. Skim milk. But only skim. Okay— 1 percent milk if you must. But nobody over the age of 4 needs the butterfat in whole milk. Wean yourself over a period of weeks by cutting back from whole to 2 percent to 1 percent or skim. Also, use 1 to 2 percent milk instead of cream in your coffee; it all adds up.

31. Lean roast beef. Fatty meats have taken a hit in the past few years, so don't eat the fat, and you don't have to eat it every day. But lean beef contains essential B vitamins, iron, and zinc. The darker the meat the better

32. Chicken. Grill it for a great entrée, then keep it around cold to munch, or throw it on a salad for an incredibly easy, vegetable-rich, low-fat meal. (Just don't eat the skin.)

33. Natural peanut butter. It's high in fat, but it's good fat, with no cholesterol. It's also high in fiber, folate, and vitamin E and can reduce the risk of cardiovascular disease. It's great on a slice of whole grain bread or a rice cake as a post-workout recovery fuel. Try it with a chicken and broccoli stir-fry. (Web site www.tastythyme.com sells a Thai Ginger and Red Pepper Peanut Butter.)

34. Cod liver oil. Researchers in Wales have found that cod liver oil can reduce enzymes associated with cartilage damage due to osteoarthritis. They gave 1,000 milligrams to patients before knee replacement surgery. Eighty-six percent of the patients produced far lower levels of the enzymes. It's a great source of vitamins A and D, but frankly, any oily fish can accomplish the same thing. There are flavored varieties. Keep it icy cold in the fridge.

35. Wine. A paper published in the *Lancet* in 1979 noted that the French, despite their notable consumption of cheese, butter, goose liver, and other fatty foods, had a lower frequency of atherosclerosis than people in other cultures who ate a lot of rich foods. The scientists put deux and deux together and decided that this "French paradox" as they called it was explained by the fact that the French washed it all down with good red wine. Same for my ancestors and relatives in sunny Italy. A 3.5-ounce glass of red wine can provide 150 milligrams of the antioxidant PCO, which protects against inflammatory degradation of the inner linings of coronary arteries. It's also rich in flavenoids.

36. Pasta. A great carb, pasta is the fuel and refuel of choice for most endurance athletes. Whole wheat and spinach pastas are great alternatives. Cut back the portions to control calories and make up the volume by adding a rainbow of vegetables like peppers, broccoli, and peas. A little olive oil, garlic, and chopped tomatoes, and you are livin' la dolce vita.

37. Cherries. These are high in antioxidants and also have anti-inflammatory properties. Recent USDA studies have shown them beneficial in easing osteoarthritis-related joint pain. They reduce blood levels of C-Reactive protein and nitric oxide, both of which are markers of inflammatory disease.

38. Grape juice and pomegranate juice. Both are high in antioxidants and very refreshing. Pomegranate juice tastes even smoother and has even more antioxidant power than red wine and green tea! Wash out those free radicals while you rehydrate.

39. Apples. High in boron (also found in broccoli, pears, grapes, and nuts), apples are important to bone and joint health. It seems that individuals with osteoarthritis have less boron in their bones and synovial fluid.

40. Smoothies. These drinks are a refreshing fun and easy way to assure adequate fruit consumption. All you need is a blender. Don't throw out older fruit; cut it up, freeze it, and mix it with some ice, low-fat yogurt, and hit the button. My health club makes "recovery shakes" that really do the job.

CHILLING OUT (STRESS REDUCTION AND ATTITUDE ADJUSTMENT)

SOMETIMES WHEN I MEET PATIENTS for the first time, even before I hear their stories or examine their ailments, I get a strong feeling that I won't be able to help them.

It's not their physical condition; it's their mindset. Whether it's stress, depression, or a seriously defeatist attitude, they have a strange, negative force that seems to emanate from every pore.

Studies show that negativity like this contributes to everything from skin rashes and hives, to high blood pressure, to immune system depletion, to less successful surgical outcomes, and to lower rates of survival following heart attacks.

We are just beginning to understand and appreciate the mechanisms that allow the mind to affect the body. Ongoing research, especially in the relatively new field of psychoneuroimmunology (PNI), is explicating the complex hormonal and biochemical triggers that alter the immune response and other physiological systems, allowing your mind and central nervous system to either give you a boost or to put you in irons.

Through most of the history of modern medicine, the mind and the body have been considered very separate domains. It's only the past few years that science and medicine have owned up to the fact that the "mind-body split," as it was called, is bogus. When dealing with medical conditions, it is more as Flanders Dunbar, MD, suggested when he said, "It is not a question of whether an illness is physical or emotional, but how much of each."

The mind-body connection also extends to athletic performance.

Many years ago, during his days as a championship bodybuilder, Arnold Schwarzenegger talked about being able to mentally direct more blood to specific muscle groups through concentration. His fellow athletes and most doctors thought he had gone around the bend, but subsequent biofeedback research has proved him right. What he had discovered on his own was the power of guided imagery, the same force that yogis have used for centuries to control heart rate, body temperature, and various other physiological effects.

To paraphrase another famous yogi—Yogi Berra—athletic performance is 90 percent physical and the other half mental. Having spent a good deal of time with professional athletes, I believe that mindset makes the difference between the consistent winners and the also-rans. Competitors' physical skills are often very close, but when the chips are down, the mind amplifies—or short circuits—talent. While you may never stand 6'9" and have the musculature of a Karl Malone, you have the same neurological capabilities that he does for focusing the mind on achievement rather than failure, repair rather than breakdown. In terms of attitude, then, we can all be champions.

For the musculoskeletal system, the most obvious mind-body connection is the role that stress plays in both acute and chronic pain. In any 6-month period, a significant percentage of adults will experience neck or low back pain, but the effect is not limited to the neck and back. Tension carried in those places is in the core, so the compensatory pain it causes can radiate almost anywhere. The distorted posture can lead to imbalances and significant problems even in the arms and legs. And then, while anxiety and stress create the tension in the first place, other emotional factors compound the damage.

Researchers at Stanford University found that patients with poor coping skills, as measured by psychological testing, were four times more likely than those with good coping skills to develop significant problems with their lower backs. In fact, the psychological test scores were far more predictive of back problems than any structural abnormalities found on MRI or other imaging! Other studies have shown that the best predictors of long-term work-related lower back disability has more to do with psychosocial factors like job performance and job satisfaction than any physical parameter tested in terms of their lower back function.

Pain can lead to disuse, which leads to atrophy, which can lead to true disability. Canadian researchers randomly selected 800 people who were painfree and followed them for a while. Of that group, those who were depressed were four times as likely as the others to develop intense or disabling pain in the neck or low back. The researchers are now doing further work to confirm what they see as the cause—passive coping mechanisms. In other words, we all have minor pains, but people who are depressed withdraw from the pain-inducing activities, or simply wish they had a better pain mecha-

nism, whereas people with a healthier state of mind stay active, which includes doing exercises that can work out the kinks and ease the pain.

In medical school, there was an unwritten rule that, if you lined up all the medical specialty areas on a spectrum, the two at the most opposite extremes were orthopaedics and psychiatry.

We bone docs were known as nuts and bolts guys, whereas psychiatry was thought of as the "pursuit of the id by the odd." We solved and manually fixed practical problems, very "hands-on"; they were lost in the murky world of existential distress.

But now we know that there are tremendous areas of overlap. So much so, that it doesn't make much sense to try to address musculoskeletal issues without seeing them in the context of emotional well-being. This is something many of my colleagues have yet to learn.

Sometimes a seemingly happy person has an injury that then leads to depression.

Injury and rehabilitation are themselves stressful—the loss of favorite activities, the boredom, the inconvenience of doctor visits, and hours with the physical therapist. So, whereas once we would try to either fix the body or fix the mind, now we work on both, in tandem.

One of the ideas we try to get across is the benefits of a positive outlook. Your mind has to change before your body can. This isn't just a superficial cliché about putting on a happy face, or even "coach talk" about motivation and a winning attitude. Studies show that optimists are actually healthier than pessimists, and that they do better on just about every other measure of well-being. Like good posture, optimism doesn't always come naturally to all of us, but we can all work on it.

Another basic concept is what psychologists call "construal," meaning that much of our reality depends on how we interpret or "construe" the facts we're confronted with. Studies show, for instance, that bronze medalists at the Olympics are much happier about their outcome than silver medalists. Why should someone who came in third feel better than someone who came in second? Well, the theory is that third place finishers are glad to be in the winner's circle at all, whereas second place finishers have that nagging feeling that "if only" they'd done something more, they might have come in first.

To some extent, that kind of nagging can be the spur for further achievement; on the other hand, it can also be a formula for never-ending dissatisfaction and long-term misery.

This idea that our attitudes create our reality jibes with the results of studies comparing people who win the lottery with people who become quadraplegics. After a brief period of being "up" about their good fortune or "down" about their very bad fortune, most people return to wherever they were before. In other words, happy people settle back into happiness, and unhappy people settle back into unhappiness. In the long run, whether they've won the lottery or become paralyzed makes no difference.

In short, a large part of the world is what we make it. It's not so much the cards you're dealt, but how you play them that counts most.

Self-image is a construal that bears importantly on fitness. In their own minds, for instance, most women can never be too thin, while most men can never be too muscular. This contributes to a variety of problems ranging from anorexia to steroid use to, once again, constant dissatisfaction and long-term misery.

Unfortunately, developing optimism and self-acceptance are complicated issues that aren't going to be resolved simply by the kind of advice I can give here. However, 30 years of mind-body medicine has given us many behavioral approaches to perhaps the most pervasive mind-body issue, which is stress.

Managing stress begins with some of the steps I've already outlined. You need to:

- Exercise regularly. Aside from all its other benefits, exercise improves mood and is a natural stress buster.

- Practice relaxation breathing. Better yet, take a restorative yoga class.

- Get 6 to 8 hours sleep a night. Restful sleep.

- Eat right and drink plenty of water! (Food affects mood and dehydration translates into dry eyes, a stiff neck, and low back pain—all associated with being stressed out.)

Whole shelves of books have been written outlining more specific stress-reduction techniques, but their three most basic themes are:

1. Short-circuiting the "fight or flight" response that needlessly revs up your body with stress hormones

2. Getting you out of your "head," meaning, shifting your focus away from a constant stream of ideas and worries produced inside your cerebral cortex

3. Putting you more in touch with the emotional and intuitive parts of your experience.

These concepts lead to several recommendations that can be of dramatic benefit for your frame. These are just the sort of thing the "tough guys" down at the bar love to laugh at, but that sissies like Olympic athletes and pro football players have discovered really work.

■ Breathe! Breathing isn't just about staying alive—as in basic air exchange in the lungs. Proper breathing is a way of filling every nook and cranny with a rejuvenating dose of oxygen. That means every cell, every muscle, every tendon, every one of those tissues we talked about undergoing constant remodeling and repair. It's also a quick way of gaining control over your stress reflexes—fight or flight— and calming yourself down. Most of us spend the day doing shallow breathing, which actually produces tension.

In yoga they call it pranayama, the Sanskrit word for breath control. They've been perfecting it for thousands of years in India, but it's actually very simple, so simple that you can do it anywhere—riding in an elevator, stuck in traffic, sitting, or standing.

1. Right where you are, straighten your spine. Close your eyes and do a couple of the neck-loosening exercises we described on page 75.

2. Begin to notice your breathing. You've been doing it since you were born, but right now actually pay close attention to it. Feel it expanding your lungs, then emptying out of your lungs.

3. As you take deeper, more conscious breaths, notice how the infusion of oxygen clears your head. Focus on the simple act of breathing and let that intense focus drive everything else from your mind.

4. Start taking even deeper, slower breaths through your nose. Fill your lungs completely full, then release the air through your mouth. Do this three or four times.

5. Breathe normally through your nose three or four times, still focusing on the oxygen coming into your body. Think about it expanding your chest and entering your blood and circulating throughout your neck and back, your forehead and temples, right down to your toes.

6. Continue taking slow, deep breaths through your nose. But now, each time you breathe, let your belly expand so that you're breathing with your diaphragm. When your lungs are completely full, hold the breath for 2 seconds (until you get this deeper breathing down, place your palms on your abdominal area and actually feel your abdomen expand).

7. Slowly release the breath through your mouth, but continue to exhale until your lungs feel completely empty. Contract your belly to force out every last ounce of air. Now wait 2 seconds.

8. Repeat the cycle with another slow, deep breath through your nose. Do three or four more cycles, then slowly open your eyes.

Chances are, your blood pressure will be lower, your head will be clearer, and just about every muscle in your body will be more relaxed. Athletes often use this to lower stress during competition.

- **Discover your stress buttons** at home, work, and school and do something about them! This means active coping, which includes talking to others to find solutions to your problems.

- **Discover what unstresses you** and make a habit of it. Play poker, build a model airplane, take a walk, see a movie, listen to your favorite tunes, play with your kids, take up the ukulele. The objective is to find something that gets you into the psychological state called "flow." Flow means a little challenge, but not too much. It's something in which your mind can become lost in the moment, fully engaged, but not striving.

- **Laugh.** Laughing has been shown to lower stress levels, relieve pain, improve sleep patterns, lower blood pressure, and boost immunity. It might even lower the risk of certain cancers. The physiological mechanism may be via the lowering of blood cortisol levels (stress hormone), as well as an increase in endorphins and growth hormones. So rent a Marx Brothers movie or call a friend who makes you laugh. Although you can't find it in any anatomy book, your "tickle bone" is probably an understimulated part of your frame. Find it.

- **Soothe yourself.** Certain repetitive sounds and images from nature, as well as mildly challenging, repetitive activities such as juggling and knitting, give the mind a rest by engaging it just enough to distract it from its usual concerns. I love to juggle, and it was surprisingly easy to learn. I've found that, in addition to being able to impress just about any child, when those balls are in the air something clicks off in my brain. I'm instantly relaxed and unable to think about more stressful things. That feeling is priceless, as was the comment by one child after watching me show my skills: "Dr. Nick, you could be a clown!" Staring into a fire, listening to the waves, and walking on the beach are not just corny, romantic things to do. At times they can be medically necessary, even if your HMO doesn't cover it. The same could be true for fly fishing or flying a kite or doing Tai Chi. I've always found that skiing, despite being very physically demanding, is actually very relaxing. More so than even harder exercise or other great vacations. Skiing (and surviving it) really forces me to take my mind off my day-to-day stresses. Again, it's that idea of engagement. The mind simply needs to rest, and to rest, it needs to play.

Rhythmic repetitive exercise like jogging and swimming will promote relaxation, too. The "runner's high" that many people experience is a real phenomenon thought to be from the release of endorphins, an opium-like substance that's released during exercise. It's one explanation for why exercise can become addictive, and why some people push it beyond what's good for them.

■ **Adopt a positive attitude.** Easier said than done, but even if you have to fake it at first, the benefits of optimism are so huge that it pays to try to learn to suspend your disbelief. My good friend Pat Croce, the maestro of positive attitude, is so upbeat that it's contagious. Read his book *I Feel Great* for a lift, and, if you can find them, hang out with people like Pat and catch their wave.

■ **Practice guided imagery.** In the same way that an aquarium in your room can lower your blood pressure, you can create images in your mind to calm yourself. Close your eyes and imagine your favorite spot at the lake or on the beach. Make up a pleasant scenario. Maybe you're fishing or making a sand castle. Maybe you're watching some little creature swim in a tide pool. Stay with the image, make it real, and your stress will ease. When you're in pain, close your eyes and imagine the sensation as a glaring light bulb. Then, gradually imagine that you have a dimmer and that you're turning down the lights bit by bit. In time, your experience of the pain should diminish.

■ **Use progressive muscle relaxation (PMR).** With PMR you basically work through every major muscle group in your body, taking inventory like a pilot in a preflight checklist, tightening and tensing each muscle group, then fully relaxing it. Unfortunately, we all keep certain muscle groups in a partially tense, partially contracted state. This not only wastes energy, ruins posture, and makes you tight, it also can develop into "trigger areas" in which a muscle locks up and causes you pain. By intentionally tightening a muscle, you can learn also to consciously relax it, by letting off the tension. You may need this in certain muscles more than others, but try it head to toe. Clench your jaw, shrug your shoulders, and tighten your fists. Arms, legs, torso, and pelvic area. Combine it with relaxation breathing and learn to turn on and off unnecessary muscle tension.

■ **Meditate or take up yoga or Tai Chi.** Meditation can have a profoundly positive effect on your blood pressure, pulse rate, breathing rate, and brain waves. It has been shown to reduce pain, depression, hostility, and anxiety as well as help a variety of medical ailments. Blood lactate levels drop. (Remember muscle soreness?) Muscles relax. You actually trigger the opposite of your body's adrenalin-filled "flight or fight" stress response, something called "the relaxation response," which is an adaptive mechanism protecting you from overstress. I've always thought of Tai Chi as "yoga in motion," and, of course, yoga is already a near-perfect form of relaxation. For a quick stressbuster during the day, try the child's pose or pillar stretch combined with relaxation breathing.

■ **Serve yourself a beverage,** and let it serve you. Tea—especially green tea—or even hot water with lemon can relax you. A glass of wine in the evening will also help you unwind as it provides those antioxidants that are so important to your health. But you definitely want to avoid coffee or other heavily caffeinated beverages around stressful times. When you have to put in those extra hours to finish the job, better to rely on hot water than a Coke or hot coffee, which, after a point, will simply make you tighten up.

Again, there is a vast literature on mind-body healing and stress reduction techniques. To learn more, I recommend reading:

Minding the Body, Mending the Mind by Joan Borysenko

The Ancestral Mind by Gregg Jacobs

Learned Optimism by Martin Seligman

Mind Body Medicine: How to Use Your Mind for Better Health by Daniel Goleman.

If depression is sometimes as issue for you, it might be time to see a therapist. You also might benefit from reading *Feeling Good* by David D. Burns, MD.

You can indeed channel your mind to help mend your body. Learn to tap this power to optimize your frame and its function.

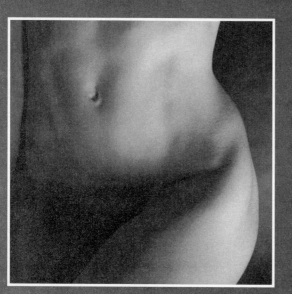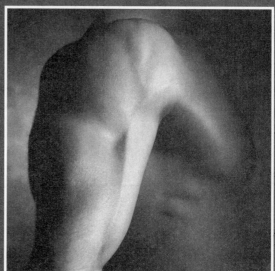

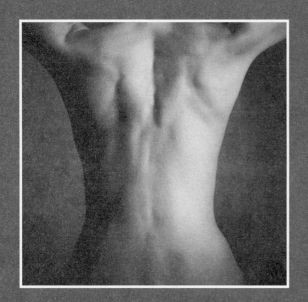

PART THREE

■

WHEN

YOUR

FRAME

FAILS

FIVE

■ ■ ■

AVOIDING INSULT ON TOP OF INJURY
(MANAGING YOUR MANAGED CARE)

WHEN A FRIEND OF MINE DECIDED IT WAS TIME TO HANG UP HIS BASKETBALL shoes and find a lower impact exercise, he bought some goggles and took up swimming, often considered the perfect activity for all-around conditioning. Next thing you know he's seeing the doctor for shoulder trouble. It seems the repetitive motion was inflaming an old injury from a bicycle accident years before. It took 6 months of physical therapy before he was back to normal.

My friend had never self-tested to monitor the old weak link. And when it re-emerged as a serious problem, he was not well-served by his general practitioner (GP), who prescribed rest and ibuprofen. When things didn't get better, the doctor

offered a cortisone injection to reduce the inflammation, but the focus was entirely on pain reduction. He never addressed the issue of impingement, or rotator-cuff weakness and imbalance. What the GP didn't consider was the way in which the old bicycle injury had distorted the action of my friend's shoulder. When he took up swimming, it was this distortion that was a setup for trouble.

When my friend at last saw an orthopaedist, the first thing the specialist pointed out was that the shoulder had become locked into a very limited range of motion, the "frozen shoulder" I talked about in Chapter 3.

Pain was one consideration, but the pain and inflammation were never going to go away until that "rusty" shoulder was "oiled," in a sense, and gradually brought back to moving in its normal arc. Also, once it became stiff, significant weakness set in and a downhill cycle began. Pain led to disuse, which led to stiffness, weakness, and ultimately more pain. Six months of physical therapy was necessary to gradually get the joint self-lubricating and moving again. That six months of therapy might not have been necessary if the weak link—the distortion from the earlier injury—had been spotted and dealt with earlier.

■ ■ ■

As I said in the Introduction, bones and joints are the number-one reason for doctor visits, accounting for 14 to 15 percent of our healthcare dollars. One of every four or five primary care visits is for a musculoskeletal problem.

Nonetheless, musculoskeletal training is less than 5 percent of the medical school curriculum. Joseph Bernstein, MD, a researcher at the University of Pennsylvania Medical School in Philadelphia, studied the results of an examination in the basics of musculoskeletal medicine given to Penn's incoming surgical and medical residents, no matter what their intended fields of specialization. Musculoskeletal problems are confronted by doctors in a number of specialties, including family practice, internal medicine, pediatrics, emergency medicine, rheumatology, and, of course, orthopaedics. Even so, 82 percent of these recent medical school graduates failed to demonstrate basic competency in the musculoskeletal examination. This is not surprising considering that orthopaedics courses or rotations were limited to an average of 2.1 weeks, with one-third of these students having had no exposure to orthopaedics at all. Those who did spend time in orthopaedics focused on a narrow range or a very superficial overview, rather than a solid grounding in the most common bone and joint problems they are likely to see in primary or emergency care. Some medical schools have even eliminated basic musculoskeletal anatomy from their curriculum.

The bottom line is that, for the number one reason that people visit the doctor in this country, nonspecialists are woefully unprepared to help them.

Adding to the problem of nonspecialists unprepared to help with bone and joint ailments is that doctors are pressed for time and pressured by HMOs to practice in a cost conscious (i.e., money-saving) way, which doesn't always lead to great interactions with patients.

In 1984, a study showed that doctors gave patients less than 20 seconds to describe their symptoms. In fact, physicians interrupted patients 18 seconds into their explanations of the problems. A follow-up study in 1999 showed improvement—physicians waited 23 seconds before interrupting patients—but that is still not what you'd call a meaningful exchange. The reports added that only 15 percent of patients fully understand what their doctors tell them, and 50 percent leave the office still uncertain of what they're supposed to do. Hurried and not terribly well-informed about bones and joints, doctors find it all too easy to say "stop what you're doing," when maybe the better idea is to modify what you're doing. For that kind of judgment call, you need a sports-oriented doctor who can give you a more informed answer.

At the same time, most general physicians have no training in the promotion and prescription of exercise, so they're not really up to the task of trying to activate the many couch potatoes who visit them each day.

What we have is really a double whammy. Doctors are needlessly slowing down or stopping the many walking wounded who usually can continue some form of exercise in a modified manner. At the same time, doctors are not able to effectively "treat" sedentary behavior, one of the leading causes of mortality in this country. I can't remake the medical establishment overnight, but I can give you some insight into healing and recovery that will help you help yourself should you become injured.

Whenever you have an acute (as opposed to chronic) soft-tissue or bone injury, you can count on your body healing in three phases:

The Reaction Phase

The Repair-Regeneration Phase

The Remodeling-Maturation Phase

THE REACTION PHASE

The body reacts to a soft-tissue injury with vascular inflammation, which means redness, swelling, and pain. It's the body's attempt to limit the extent of injury, remove damaged tissue from the wound, and initiate tissue repair.

Almost instantly, whenever blood vessels and lymphatic channels are injured, blood and plasma seep into the interstitial space, collecting with cellular debris and damaged tissue. To keep this swelling from getting out of hand, as well as to reduce blood loss, the blood vessels constrict, blood platelets pile up at the site of injury, and the blood begins to coagulate. This appears as a bruise or as a swollen lump of blood called a hematoma.

This period when your body shuts down the inflow of blood lasts only a few minutes, after which the vessels dilate once again, bringing fresh blood flow back into the injured area. Mast cells and basophils release histamine, which causes a further increase in blood flow. Platelets, in addition to their role in helping to form a clot, provide serotonin, which works along with histamine to make blood vessels more permeable, which makes it easier for the white blood cells that protect us from foreign organisms to pass through the blood vessel walls and congregate at the site of injury. Other white cells called macrophages (which means, essentially, big eaters) also congregate to remove cellular debris caused by the injury. They're the garbage patrol, there to take out the trash.

Understanding what's going on in these first moments helps to explain why prompt first aid treatment to relatively minor injuries can have a dramatic effect on your degree of discomfort. And that's one of the reasons why the pros seem to recover more quickly than you and me. They have immediate, at-the-moment-of-injury access to top-notch medical care and our medical bag of tricks.

THE REPAIR-REGENERATION PHASE

A couple of days after injury, while the now clotted swelling around the wound provides a certain degree of stability, a second wave of cells called fibroblasts begin the process of wound repair by producing new collagen.

Special enzymes begin to further degrade damaged tissue. At the same time, tiny blood vessels proliferate and connect to form a new capillary bed.

About 4 days after injury, the new collagen secreted by the fibroblasts begins to offset the collagen degradation that has taken place, which adds further to the wound's tensile strength. At the same time, though, the wound begins to contract, which accounts for some of the stiffness in ligaments and muscles following injury.

THE REMODELING-MATURATION PHASE

The remodeling process begins as early as 3 weeks following injury, and then, in many instances, it continues for a year or more.

Collagen also remodels itself, influenced by the kind of mechanical load imposed on the injured area. The collagen fibers reorient themselves along the lines of tensile force. But when Hemingway talked about being strong at the broken places, he was not talking about orthopaedic injuries. The ultimate tensile strength of scars may be as much as 30 percent less than that of the original tissue.

THE THREE PHASES OF BONE HEALING

Most fractures can be easily diagnosed with a simple x-ray. Some, more subtle ones, require special imaging studies such as a bone scan or MRI to see the fracture line or crack. This is especially true of overuse-related stress fractures that notoriously show up as normal on x-rays early in the process.

Bone injuries also heal according to a three-part schedule. But unlike soft tissue healing in which there's always a tradeoff with formation of some sort of scar tissue, bone actually heals as good as new.

When a bone is fractured, inflammation begins immediately. Bleeding from the fracture site and surrounding soft tissues once again creates a swelling, or hematoma, as well as fibrin clot. Again, the blood supply is temporarily disrupted, but within hours it increases. It's the blood vessels supplying bone with nutrients that allows it to self-repair. The abnormal movement of damaged bone ends, along with hemorrhage from damaged blood vessels and nerve irritation, is why it hurts so much to break an arm or a leg.

After this period of inflammation, the repair phase begins. Osteoclasts begin to eat away at fractured bone surfaces, removing debris. New cells drawn to the site of injury give rise to osteoblasts, the builder cells that secrete new osteoid, the organic matrix.

Capillaries grow among the bone cells, forming a tissue called callus that bridges the gap between the broken ends. The new bone that is produced is relatively weak and is converted to lamellar or mature bone during later remodeling.

With an acute bone injury, remodeling begins during the middle of the repair phase and continues for months or even several years, long after the fracture has clinically healed. Remodeling allows the bone to assume its normal configuration and shape based on the stresses to which it is exposed. Throughout this process, woven bone formed during the repair phase is replaced with lamellar bone. Fracture healing is complete when the marrow is repopulated with the cells that differentiate to become new blood cells. We use x-rays to monitor fracture healing, and the fracture is usually well healed before the "fracture line" disappears on film.

Fractures usually heal like clockwork, but not always. Certain bones like the tibia (or shin), humerus (or upper arm), clavicle (or collarbone), and navicular (both the hand and foot) can take longer at times, a process called "delayed union." At other times the repair process completely shuts down before healing occurs, called a "non-union." These fracture-healing problems are more common in adults, smokers, and those with more serious comminuted (shattered, not a clean break) fractures or open (skin disrupted with a wound over the bone) fractures. Newer repair techniques and the use of "bone stimulators" (small, battery-powered, painless devices worn over the fracture area) have made these fracture difficulties less common.

COPING WITH INJURY

Doctors use the acronym RICE (rest, ice, compression and elevation) to highlight the first steps you should take with most minor musculoskeletal injuries. When we say "rest," we actually mean "relative rest." The injured part needs to be protected from further harm, and in the very early phases after injury, especially the acute period where swelling predominates, complete and total rest may be appropriate. Shortly after that, and under the guidance of your doctor or trainer, you should start controlled, protected activity to enhance both healing and recovery. The key is to find activities that don't interfere with or set back the injury, promote better healing, and also allow you to maintain conditioning while the injury heals.

Ice is the second RICE step. The immediate application of ice or a cold compress obviously reduces temperature, but it also reduces inflammation, metabolic rate, circulation, and muscle spasm. It may also limit the extent of secondary injury resulting from tissues not getting enough oxygen.

As with compression and elevation, don't wait to ice. The sooner you apply these remedies, the better the results.

Cold suppresses the inflammatory re-

sponse by reducing the release of histamine and by decreasing capillary permeability, which helps reduce bleeding and the secondary formation of edema. It decreases pain by reducing the threshold of afferent nerve endings, which, by reducing the sensitivity of muscle spindles, helps to decrease muscle spasms.

With the pros, we use a cryocuff, which is like a boot or glove that applies continuous cold, compressed air and is very effective in preventing and reducing swelling. But you don't need anything so fancy. A bag of frozen peas will do the trick, but I prefer crushed ice in a plastic bag or baggie.

First, moisten a thin washcloth in cold water and wring it out. Place it over the injured part and then apply the ice bag and hold it in place with an elastic bandage. Don't exceed 20 to 30 minutes and repeat every hour if needed.

Another alternative is to use ice massage. This works best over superficial, bony areas such as the elbow, hand, or foot. Fill a polystyrene cup to the brim and leave it in the freezer. Once the water is frozen, you can hold the cup (so your fingers won't go numb) and massage the affected area for 5 to 10 minutes. Be very careful with frozen gel packs, though. Unlike ice, they will get as cold as your freezer and thus can cause frostbite when placed directly on the skin, especially when first removed from the freezer. Use the washcloth technique already described to protect your skin.

The third RICE element, compression, not only limits swelling but adds to the penetration of cooling and the effectiveness of ice by discouraging further leakage from the capillary beds into the spaces between the tissues.

The last RICE step, elevation, puts gravity to work for you, reducing swelling by decreasing blood flow to the injured area. But an inch or two doesn't get the job done. By elevation I mean higher than your head or heart, which is the part that most people miss. It is not enough to prop your sprained ankle up on an ottoman. Also, the sooner you get it elevated after injury, the less swelling there will be. The less swelling, the quicker the recovery.

Some people look to heat instead of ice. At times, this is the right idea. Heat provides for muscle relaxation. This occurs by relieving pain, producing sedation, and decreasing muscle tension. Increased temperature increases the elasticity and decreases the viscosity of connective tissue. Heat also has been shown to inhibit muscle spindles, thereby decreasing muscle sensitivity to stretch, and, consequently, muscle spasm. That's why heat may be helpful prior to performing stretching exercises.

But I recommend using heat only after you are over the acute swelling phase, unless you are under the care of a physical therapist or athletic trainer who knows how to use heat and ice simultaneously ("contrast baths") in the earlier phases. We're not absolutely certain why heat eases pain, but it may be due to the so-called "gate control" theory of pain modulation. The idea is that a nonpainful stimulus, such as heat, blocks the transmission of the painful stimulus.

Another physiologic effect of heat is an increase in local metabolic rate. This leads to the production of metabolites and thus additional heat, which can facilitate lymphatic drainage. Heat also can control subacute or chronic inflammation, encourage tissue healing, and reduce edema and bruising.

Superficial heating agents include moist heat packs and a warm whirlpool; deep heating agents include ultrasound. Compared with the effects of cold, heat can be more penetrating and longer lasting.

That said, ice or a cold compress on a troubled joint is the right idea after physical activity. If a joint is painful, and you're going to do range-of-motion exercises, ice is the right idea. If stiffness is what's limiting your motion, then heat is more appropriate. Heat is good for more chronic ailments, especially if there is stiffness or muscle tightness involved.

In general, if it's swollen, use ice; if it's tight and stiff, try heat. Some of this involves experimentation, since some individuals respond more to one than the other, but they are both great, inexpensive modalities.

REMEDIES FOR PAIN AND INFLAMMATION

Nonsteroidal anti-inflammatory drugs (NSAIDs) include aspirin, ibuprofen, indomethacin, naproxen, and newer COX-2 alternatives such as Bextra and Celebrex. They decrease inflammation in traumatized tissue, and they decrease the pain associated with injury and possibly stiffness as well. They control the chronic inflammatory symptoms in overuse injuries, especially those stemming from degeneration caused by previous injuries. They can also help limit the soft-tissue necrosis resulting from the "inflammatory overshoot" following acute trauma.

A word of caution, however. NSAIDs may interfere with bone healing, joint surface re-growth, and tendon repairs. And all NSAIDs share a potential to cause abdominal problems like peptic bleeding and gastrointestinal ulceration and interfere with platelet function, as well as liver toxicity. Vioxx was recently withdrawn from the marketplace because of cardiovascular complications associated with its use, something that has also prompted a more cautious use of the other COX-2 alternatives such as Bextra and Celebrex.

The decision to use an NSAID for sports-related injuries, then, should be driven by the need for anti-inflammatory relief, rather than for pain relief alone, and there should be time limits on use, something best determined by your physician and the nature of your injury.

Despite all the advertising claims, studies have never shown a clear superiority of one NSAID over another in treating soft-tissue injuries or joint inflammation. Some individuals seem to respond better to one than another, so if one NSAID is not working for you, try something else. But never mix and match. By taking more than one, you decrease the effectiveness of either one, and you may also be setting yourself up for other medical complications.

Start your NSAID as soon as possible after injury and continue only for several days. Once the injury has moved into the matura-

tion phase, the NSAID offers little advantage, so you should discontinue its use. Any residual pain can be controlled with acetaminophen (Tylenol and other brands) as well as the use of ice or heat.

NSAIDs have not been shown to contribute significantly to the restoration of normal tissue function following injury or hasten a return to participation in sports.

CORTICOSTEROIDS

Corticosteroids, such as cortisone, hydrocortisone, prednisone, and triamcinolone, have a far greater anti-inflammatory power; however, they also share a far greater frequency of serious complications.

Overdependence on corticosteroids is all part of the old school, play-through-the-numbed-pain of *North Dallas Forty*. Corticosteroids act to suppress inflammation by inhibiting capillary dilation, inflammatory cell migration, and tissue edema, but they also inhibit capillary and fibroblast proliferation, as well as collagen synthesis during the repair phase of healing. They should never be used immediately before a competitive event or if an infection is present. Too many athletes over the years have seriously injured themselves after having their pain numbed by injections just to get them back on the field or court, which is not the same thing as having intact tissue structure or function. When used properly, and for the right indications—to help reduce pain and improve function, allowing the patient to participate in rehabilitation—steroid shots are safe and effective. However, corticosteroids can damage tendons and ligaments, a factor that has to be weighed against the potential therapeutic effect. They may also cause tissue atrophy and localized loss of skin pigmentation.

Injections should be done only after other conservative treatment approaches such as rest and exercise have failed. In general, no more than three steroid injections should be given to any one joint or tendon area in a given year. They should never be used in lieu of good preventive rehabilitation.

Steroid injections sometime lure a patient into resuming normal activity instead of looking for root causes, i.e., faulty training or technique. All too often this leads to further injury.

Because corticosteriods can tear down tissue, they usually should not be used following acute trauma, and if you have had an injection, usually plan for 10 to 14 days off from heavier use of the involved area (especially days off from whatever got you into trouble in the first place). Corticosteroids should never be directly injected into the tendon but rather into the surrounding tissue where they can bathe the tendon. Certain tendons, such as the infrapatellar tendon below the kneecap and the Achilles tendon, should never be injected because of the likelihood of full tendon rupture.

ULTRASOUND

If you see a physical therapist to help rehabilitate an injury, he may apply ultrasound. Scientific understanding of the underlying mechanisms is fairly primitive, but low-intensity ultrasound during bone repair appears to accelerate healing. In soft tissues, ultrasound is believed to reduce edema, pain, and muscle spasms.

The lower intensity sound waves of ultrasound also alter cell membrane permeability to increase the flow of metabolites and ions, especially calcium. Ultrasound draws cells that can expedite tissue repair to the injury site. During the proliferative phase of inflammation, ultrasound increases the entry of calcium ions that signal the cells to enhance their metabolic machinery to a reparative mode. Ultrasound enhances wound contraction, the growth of new blood vessels, and collagen production, which leads to increased tensile strength.

ELECTRICAL STIMULATION AND H-WAVE

Your therapist may also employ electric fields, which can modify the orientation of soft-tissue collagen fibers.

The body has natural electric currents that travel along nerves, as well as transmembrane voltages in the cells. But there are also measurable currents in skin and other cells that facilitate wound repair. A wound, which is a break in the skin, muscle, or tendon, produces what is essentially a short circuit in these electric lines.

Providing therapeutic electric stimulation to the wounded tissue attempts to mimic the body's natural healing response. Electrical stimulation allows sodium ions to enter the outer cells of the epithelium, then diffuse to other cells. Positively charged ions such as fibroblasts and activated neutrophils migrate toward the negative electrode (the cathode). Meanwhile, negatively charged ions and cells such as epidermal cells, macrophages and neutrophils migrate toward the positive electrode (the anode). Electrical stimulation also inhibits bacterial growth, improves blood flow, reduces edema, stimulates fibroplasia (the growth of fibroblast cells), and improves wound tensile strength.

Different electrical stimulation devices have different functions, which are determined by various physiological factors. By varying the intensity and/or duration of the electrical impulse, or the waveform itself, you can get different results at the tissue and cellular level. Some devices, like transcutaneous electrical nerve stimulation (TENS) specifically target the sensory nerves and are used for pain control only. High-volt galvanic stimulation is used not only for pain relief but also to generate muscle contractions, which are useful to prevent atrophy and reduce swelling.

H-Wave is a unique electrical stimulation device with a waveform that has numerous capabilities. The current can be varied depending on rehabilitation goals. It not only reduces the pain of acute and chronic injuries but is terrific for nerve-related pain. It also enhances wound healing, especially in chronic, slow healing, compromised wounds, as well as in managing diabetic wounds and diabetic neuropathy. The "lymphatic pump" encouraged by the electrical impulses, in conjunction with the associated muscle contractions, reduces swelling and inflammation, which results in pain reduction and quicker recovery.

Also fluid shifts and changes in tissue pH optimize the cellular environment for recovery. It's no wonder we're always slapping H-Wave units on our injured Philadelphia 76ers and dancers.

Gary Vitti, the highly respected and innovative longtime trainer for the Los Angeles Lakers, feels that H-Wave is indispensable in keeping his guys above the rim. Jeffrey Spencer, DC, a chiropractor who works with Lance Armstrong and the United States Postal Service Pro Cycling Team, says he wouldn't leave home without it. It also enhances muscle recovery after grueling workouts, which is why Lance uses it frequently during the Tour de France.

Muscle stimulation not only enhances recovery but also prevents muscle loss and atrophy around injuries. It's the perfect way to start rebuilding strength for those who are in too much pain or are too weak to exercise following injury, surgery, or immobilization. I've also found it very useful in many acute and chronic pain syndromes, especially tendinitis and tendinosis.

PHONOPHORESIS AND IONTOPHORESIS

Corticosteroid creams or other pain-reducing gels can be used in conjunction with ultrasound (phonophoresis) or electrical stimulation (iontophoresis) to drive those molecules to deeper tissues in order to reduce pain and inflammation, as well as to enhance healing at deeper tissue levels. These modalities are used by physical therapists and athletic trainers very frequently in the rehabilitation setting, especially with tendinitis.

BONE STIMULATORS

Your bones also sense mechanical forces and convert them into electrical impulses at the bone surface and cellular levels. Following the fracture of a long bone, osteoblasts can be directed by an electrical signal to the concave or compression bone surface. This site of local electronegativity becomes the site of greatest bone deposition. Meanwhile, osteoclasts digest bone on the electropositive side of the fracture, which is equivalently the convex or tension side. The remodeling phase of bone healing is essentially an accelerated form of normal bone turnover that culminates in the restoration of normal shape, strength, and function. Again, ultrasound and electrical (even electromagnetic) stimulation can both accelerate and enhance fracture healing and remodeling.

ACUPUNCTURE

We still have much to learn about why and how acupuncture works, but the best explanation to date, confirmed by MRI studies, is that the tiny needles, placed in exactly the right points in the body, decrease blood flow to the brain. When there's less blood to a certain area, that area of the brain quiets down, apparently releasing endorphins, the brain's natural pain-relieving and comforting chemicals. Acupuncture is a great therapy for individuals with chronic neck or back pain, acute or chronic nerve pain, or in other instances in which traditional Western methods have failed. Other people just can't tolerate medications such as NSAIDs because of allergies or other medical issues, and for them acupuncture is a welcome alternative.

THERAPEUTIC EXERCISE

As I've said before, exercise itself can be a therapeutic medicine for tendons, ligaments, and muscles. When put under load, collagen fibers may transmit physical signals that induce changes in cellular metabolism and the synthesis of proteoglycans and matrix. Both tension and pressure modify cell synthesis in tendon and articular cartilage, and these changes can hasten the return of structural integrity. During healing, you get a better quality scar if you rely on controlled movement rather than immobilization.

GOOD NUTRITION

High-quality calories really count when you're on the comeback trail. Breaking your femur (or thigh bone) may increase basal metabolism of around 20 percent as your body gears up to repair the injured bone. This means that a female athlete who might burn 1,600 calories during a typical, nonworkout day could see her caloric requirements shoot up to 2,000 calories because of the bone break. However, the changes in nutrient requirements in response to an injury are not simply a matter of increased caloric needs; various parts of the body have unique nutritional demands, and the optimal nutritional plan to restore an injury to cartilage might differ from the best scheme for repairing muscles or nerves. You must also weigh into the equation the drop in calories burned through exercise and training, now limited by injury.

If you have a bone injury, you may need to bump up your daily calcium intake to 1,500 milligrams. In general, when you're recovering from injury, your body needs more calories just to fuel the repair process. So go ahead and eat—and don't worry about gaining weight while you're on the sidelines, especially if you can find creative ways to safely stay active. The worst thing you can do, both to retard healing and to invite subsequent injury, is to deprive your body of the nutrients it needs. Just be sure you get high-quality calories, not naked ones.

During recovery, you should increase your protein to 100 to 120 grams a day. You need 80 to 100 grams a day just to maintain your muscles and soft tissues, and that's before adding on the task of healing.

Some extra vitamin A can help rebuild your tissues, including skin, so pile on the leafy green vegetables, yellow and orange fruits and vegetables, and fortified skim milk. Make sure you're getting enough vitamin C, which combats free radicals and helps your body make the collagen you need to repair soft tissues.

MANAGING YOUR MANAGED CARE

Prevention of injury is our number-one goal, but once things go wrong it's important that you get:

- Early and accurate diagnosis

- Early and proper treatment

- Education about your condition

- Full functional rehabilitation and recovery

- A program of prevention so the injury doesn't happen again

Unfortunately, in our overly complex healthcare system, some of these steps get short shrift. Delays in care are common, but sometimes this is the patient's fault. You wait, hoping things will get better on their own, or you ignore the warnings and continue "playing through the pain." At other times it's the system that's at fault. Maybe you can't get an appointment. Most people start with their primary care physician, which is fine, but we've already discussed their limitations in evaluating and treating your frame malfunctions. What you need is a primary care physician who knows his or her limitations and is willing, when necessary, to refer you to a specialist earlier rather than later. You may have to speak up to get what you want, especially if your situation seems more serious to you, or if your recovery is not going as well as planned.

To find a board certified orthopaedic surgeon in your area, check www.aaos.org. To find one with more credentials in the sports medicine world, check www.sportsmed.org. Other useful Web sites for your frame include www.drnick.com (my site) and www.ortho info.aaos.org.

Many orthopaedic surgeons subspecialize, focusing on just one body part such as the knee, shoulder, hand, or spine. I personally think that if all you do is one thing, like knees, day in and day out, you get better at it. You may want to find a subspecialist for your "weak link," especially if it's more serious, complicated, requires surgery, or is a recurrent problem.

There are other physicians who can help with your frame. Rheumatologists are not surgeons, but they specialize in arthritis, especially the unusual or chronic forms. They also are often good with fibromyalgia. Physiatrists are medical doctors with specialty training in rehabilitation.

Some primary care physicians take an extra year or two of training in nonsurgical aspects of sports medicine and are very good at dealing with sports injuries and rehabilitation. This emerging field is called primary care sports medicine.

Then there are physical therapists, athletic trainers, chiropractors, and podiatrists, who are all part of the frame team. Physical therapists and athletic trainers are worth their weight in gold in terms of rehabilitation and prevention of sports injuries. And podiatrists can help with nagging foot and ankle issues and fabricate orthotics when indicated.

Many of my orthopaedic colleagues still cringe when I say the word chiropractor, but this bias comes from years of misinformation and turf battles, something we need to move beyond if we're going to put the patient first.

Many individuals do indeed benefit from chiropractic care. I was first introduced to the benefits of chiropractic care by professional dancers, an appreciation later reinforced by working with high-level athletes, who sometimes bring their chiropractors with them on the road. Our 76ers' chiropractor, Dr. Neal Liebman, has hands of gold and is probably the hardest-working member of our medical staff during game time. Chiropractors are especially valuable for mechanical neck and back problems that don't involve nerve damage, as well as preventive mobilization techniques for higher-level athletes. I do not recommend chiropractic care for medical conditions such as diabetes, high blood pressure, or other ailments better served by traditional medicine.

A DIFFERENT KIND OF SECOND OPINION

Another thing I've learned from years working with dancers is that so many sports injuries, especially the nagging, chronic, recurrent overuse variety, are rooted not in a single obvious injury, but in technical flaws you bring to the event. I can get most injured dancers better, but often it also takes a consultation with a ballet master skilled in technique to find the subtle, biomechanical bad habit that is the root of the dancer's problem.

Instead of recommending more doctors, more MRIs, or more cortisone shots, I often recommend that you work with a knowledgeable coach, trainer, or instructor to see why you're getting into trouble. Tennis or golfer's elbow—take a lesson. Sure I can inject your elbow with some cortisone, and you'd feel better. But if you go out and play with that faulty stroke, or wrong size grip, you'll be back pretty soon. Same for cycling injuries. Go to a good bike shop for an evaluation. Minor changes on your bike frame could mean avoiding surgery on a much more expensive human frame.

Part of my healthcare team in getting runners back on the road are the terrific staff (all runners) at Bryn Mawr Running Company, who will not only review your running program but will help you find the right shoes and inserts for your problem. For finding the technical issues at the root of so many athletic ailments, there are now centers that specialize in biomechanical analysis of athletes, using high-speed computerized video. This has helped many pitchers with bum shoulders and runners with recurrent overuse injuries. You might never expect a doctor to be saying this, but in medicine, we don't know everything. Sometimes we have to tap into the knowledge of others.

FIX ME, DOC!

In this country we have tremendous resources to keep you in tip-top shape—the best healthcare in the world. The wealthy travel from all over the globe to the United States for medical care, but that's only half the equation. You need to do your part in your own recovery. Often I find that individuals can do more for themselves than I can do for them. Physicians and other health professionals can point you in the right direction, or patch you up when needed, but ultimately you're in charge of your own health. The patients who do best assume their share of responsibility, following through with recommended exercise, diet, and medication. The same is true for the FrameWork Plan. It gives you the tools you need, but ultimately, it's up to you to put them to work.

SIX

■ ■ ■

A Scar Is Born:
When Surgery Is the Answer

I MENTIONED EARLIER THAT DOCTORS ARE NOT KNOWN FOR THEIR COMMUNICA-tion skills. Well, frankly, surgeons are the worst.

A truly great orthopaedist, one of my instructors during my residency training, said to me one day after he'd retired from the Operating Room (OR), "I never realized how interesting my patients are." Back when he was operating, he was notorious for interacting with his patients as little as possible. When we were residents observing his patient interviews, we'd have to leave the room to keep from laughing. He'd breeze in, nod to the slightly stunned patient on the examining table, give a quick look at the knee or hip, then call out to his nurse, "Barb, set 'em up for surgery!" A handshake, goodbye, and that was it.

Surgeons have learned to reach out to their patients a bit more over the past 20 years, but anyone contemplating surgery needs to realize that when it comes to getting the information they need, and then making good decisions based on that information, the responsibility falls squarely on their own shoulders. Some people find it more comforting to fall into a childlike role, relying on the highly trained authority figure to know what's best. But it's your body and your health, and the issues are rarely so clear cut that an "objec-tive" professional can make the right choice for you. When doctors are in training, they learn how to operate. As they gain experi-ence, they learn when and—more impor-tantly—when *not* to operate. Not all surgeons reach that final plateau of judg-ment, however. Surgery often involves trade-offs and tough choices, and while the professionals can supply you with technical information and statistics, nobody but you can make the judgments about what you really want.

Even more than that, you need to realize just how much a successful surgical result de-

■ ■ ■

193

pends on *you*. Getting the body put back together properly is the surgeon's responsibility, but that only carries you so far. It's how the body functions after healing that counts, and that outcome depends on the weeks or even months you spend in rehabilitation. A great physical therapist can guide you, but the critical factor is your compliance. Even though it may hurt, and even though you think you're going to pull things apart, you often have to start motion and stretching *very* early after a procedure to avoid scar tissue that will impede movement. Sometimes surgeons underplay the value of physical therapy, even as they're prescribing it, which undercuts patient compliance. But let me be clear: The game is really won or lost in your compliance at home, taking the time to do all the seemingly boring, yet essential, exercises your doctor or physical therapist assigns you, and doing them right.

Expectations can drive outcomes, and sometimes patients are counting on "good as new" as their outcome, when in actuality, "better" is all that can be expected. And the technical outcome as the doctor sees it, looking at the x-ray, or how much your knee bends or how tight your new ligament is, doesn't necessarily correlate 100 percent with the functional improvement as you see it, or as you hoped it would be. The result: happy surgeon, unhappy patient. Arthritis can result from any joint injury, and surgery may not be able to help that. Not all doctors are good at spelling these things out up front, before cutting, and patients need to be persistent until everything is clearly spelled out.

It's also true that patients are often nervous and sometimes don't absorb or remember.

Often just hearing the word "surgery" is enough to overwhelm some people, and nothing else that is said or done really sticks.

The questions that need to be resolved in that first conversation about surgery, or shortly thereafter, include:

- Is this procedure necessary or is it merely advisable?

- Is this just a little pain I can live with, or am I going to harm myself if I don't get this fixed?

- How much will it improve the situation, a little or a lot? Ask for a percentage.

- Can it wait? What problems will arise if I do wait?

- What's the recovery time?

- How long will I be out of work? Out of sports and leisure activities?

- Are there regional variations in techniques or in how or how often this procedure is done?

- Is this really the best surgeon for the job?

- How many such procedures does he or she do a year?

- Will I need general anesthesia, or will a nerve block do the trick?

- Will I need extensive therapy?

Be careful of a surgeon who appears too knife-happy or unwilling to discuss alternate nonsurgical options. Sometimes surgery is the only answer, but not often. As much as I prefer subspecialists, and think you are more likely to get a better result with a knee or shoulder guru, statistics show that for certain conditions, subspecialists are more likely to operate than others.

Take two individuals with the same spine problem living in different regions of our country. One will have 10 times the likelihood of undergoing spine surgery than the other. The variation may be more about how many fellowship trained (i.e., extra training in a subspecialty) spine surgeons practice in one area versus the other. Despite having no difference in the incidence of spine problems, the rate of spine surgery in the United States is dramatically higher than anywhere else in the world. This regional variation and surgical rates for similar conditions extends beyond orthopaedic surgery and includes cardiac and other surgeries. Are some surgeons over-operating or others under-operating? We don't yet know, but quality care should not vary that much. If there is any doubt in your personal case, get a second opinion.

Ask for printouts or Web site recommendations. Many doctors supply printed instructions. In my office, I have a nurse practitioner who follows up with patients to make sure they're clear on everything that we've discussed. I encourage questions and dialogue. Making the diagnosis is often easy; making the connection is the real challenge.

You may want to take a tape recorder to your consultation or bring a friend to take notes. And don't be afraid to ask questions and to ask for a repeat if you're not sure. Sometimes doctors are like a caller rattling off his phone number into your answering machine. The number is the critical part of the message, but they race through it because they know it so well. You don't know it, and you can miss it. Ask your doctor to slow down, be explicit, and clarify in simple terms anything you're not sure about. Ask to speak with other patients who had similar conditions.

You also need an honest and open discussion of which tests are necessary. These days, many people assume that you have to have an MRI to get complete care. The distinction, however, is actually much more subtle than that. MRI scans represent a tremendous advancement, but they are not always needed, and the MRI has not taken the place of the x-ray. In my opinion, MRIs are probably over-ordered. The real issue is whether the scan, lab tests, or any study is needed for the diagnosis and if the results of the tests will change treatment at this time.

Everyday I see patients who have had knee MRIs (no x-rays yet) ordered by their well-meaning primary care physicians. They arrive with their MRIs and the diagnosis of a "torn cartilage," expecting an easy fix with a simple arthroscopic procedure. When I take a standing x-ray and their films show severe arthritis, the MRIs and "torn cartilage" results really don't matter. A simple x-ray had the full answer; the MRIs were not only unnecessary but misleading. The arthritis is well beyond any simple arthroscopic procedure, and they need to either live with the arthritis or consider a major knee joint replacement. Imagine their surprise and that of their referring doctors. In days past, defensive medicine drove a lot of docs to write unnecessary prescriptions. Now it also drives many unnecessary MRIs.

People say that good judgment comes

from experience, and that experience comes from bad judgment. For doctors, the practice of surgery is a lifetime of learning. As science and technology move on, we have to keep up with it, learning to do things we were never taught in our residency programs.

But patients need to know that mistakes do happen. In orthopaedics, the classic mistake is operating on the wrong side, meaning the wrong knee or ankle. It doesn't happen often, but it does happen, which is why the American Academy of Orthopaedic Surgeons (AAOS) has instituted a "sign your site" program. Accordingly, every patient should insist that his surgeon come for a preoperative visit before going into the OR and sign his or her name or initial on the site where the work is to be done, while you are still awake and alert. For spine surgery, make sure the surgeon takes an intraoperative x-ray to assure the correct level for surgery.

In choosing your surgeon for a particular procedure, you should know that the best results are associated with the doctors and the hospitals that do that particular procedure every day, week after week. This means that you should look for *the* knee specialist or *the* shoulder specialist in your area.

You'll probably begin with a referral from your friends or general practitioner, but www.bestdoctors.com is a good place to go for further information as is the Web site for the American Academy of Orthopaedic Surgeons(www.aaos.org).

You can also call the public relations department of your local sports franchise or college team and ask who they use for knees, ankles, or other body parts. Again, you want the surgeon who does this procedure every day. If you are a dancer, call your local professional ballet company.

Organizations like the AAOS are working diligently to improve the care you get and make it as safe as possible. For excellent information on how to navigate your musculoskeletal care when needed, visit www.orthoinfo.aaos.org and search "Patient Safety."

THE BRIGHT SIDE

If you're an athlete or just an active individual, it is likely that at some point you may face surgery for your frame. Musculoskeletal or orthopaedic surgical procedures are among the most common operations performed these days. The rates are rising in part because of the explosion of sports and activity-related injuries, along with an aging population that includes the beat-up baby boomers with "boomeritis."

Fortunately, as surgical rates rise, incisions get smaller, techniques get better, and recovery is more rapid with far greater likelihood of returning to a full active lifestyle. You are an integral player in your healthcare team, and if you participate in your own care, things always go better.

Ask questions, follow instructions, and you will be on the road to recovery. Meanwhile, in terms of musculoskeletal prevention and treatment, the future has never been brighter, as you'll see in the next chapter.

SEVEN

■ ■ ■

"CHICKEN SOUP FOR THE KNEE" AND OTHER GLIMPSES INTO THE FUTURE

AT THE UNIVERSITY OF PENNSYLVANIA IN PHILADELPHIA, A TEAM OF RESEARCHERS led by H. Lee Sweeney, PhD, injected a synthetic gene into a mouse. This altered gene carried instructions to produce more of the protein that makes muscles grow and helps them repair themselves when they've been damaged. As a result, this mouse did some serious bulking up. His muscle mass grew to 60 percent greater than that of a normal mouse. In terms of performance, the mouse could run up and down a ladder with three times his body weight strapped on his back.

Genetic engineering has been around since the 1970s, but after 30 years of development, it's getting ready for prime time. The Human Genome Project has mapped the entire genetic inheritance, and work now being done on mice will soon be done on humans.

What Dr. Sweeney and his team did was isolate the gene that codes for insulin-like growth factor 1 (IGF-1). They inserted this gene into a virus that had been stripped of its disease-causing ability, then injected the virus—with its synthetic gene—into the muscle tissue of the mouse. Once injected, the new gene began to reproduce itself inside the mouse's cells.

Fast forward a few years, and the hope is to use this same technique to slow the muscle deterioration brought on by muscular dystrophy, or even from normal aging. This could greatly reduce the number of hip fractures in the elderly and give people much greater mobility in their later years.

But with a different spin, the same research might be able to produce a pitcher with a 120 mph fastball. And because this pitcher's muscle would no longer lose IGF-1 with age, he might be able to keep throwing heat into his fifties, or sixties, or beyond. For those nagging, recurrent muscle pulls, recovery would be only a shot away.

The *New England Journal of Medicine*

■ ■ ■

has reported the story of a baby born with a double dose of a genetic mutation known to produce immense strength in cattle. This little guy showed up in the newborn unit with bulging, well-defined muscles—a sort of mini Arnold. His mother had been a champion sprinter; his grandfather had been a construction worker notable for being able to lift 330-pound curbstones. It seems that the family's innate strength was due to their reduced level of a substance called myostatin. When doctors did genetic tests, they found that the mother had one nonfunctioning copy of the gene for the substance. In her super strong baby, both copies of the gene were nonfunctioning; he was getting no myostatin at all. Now researchers are working to develop drugs that will block myostatin in order to help people with muscular dystrophy or other illnesses in which muscles waste away. Researchers acknowledge, however, that their research inevitably will find its way into the world of athletics.

The specter of genetically enhanced super athletes is very real, so much so that the International Olympic Committee held a symposium on gene manipulation at the Cold Spring Harbor Laboratory on Long Island, New York. In fact, Professor Sweeney has been contacted by several athletes who heard about his research and are ready to volunteer to receive a new IGF-1 gene. But in the athletes' enthusiasm for bulking up, they may be overlooking certain risks. The scientists have already genetically enhanced a fly's flight muscles so that they were 300 percent stronger. The only problem was the fly couldn't get off the ground.

DESIGNER GENES AND THE PARTS DEPARTMENT

Meanwhile, other researchers are investigating less dramatic ways of using genetic engineering to deal with problems like anterior cruciate ligament (ACL) tears and stress fractures. An early report from the University of Pittsburgh suggests that recovery from sports-related injuries involving slow-healing tissues can be significantly sped up through gene therapy that enhances growth factors. Someday in the not too distant future, treatment for injured tendons, cartilage, or ligaments will be an injection. It won't repair the worn-out structure; it will regenerate it—like a salamander regrowing its tail.

A hundred years ago, modern medicine began to make great advances in healing and repair. More recently, doctors and public health officials opened up a new front in trying to change individual behaviors to prevent illness. The next great leap forward is going to be medicine that is not merely reparative, or preventative, but regenerative.

The broadest front in the movement toward regenerative medicine is stem-cell research. Stem cells are structures that have not yet differentiated into skin cells, muscle cells, or soft tissue cells. This means that they still have the potential to become almost anything. By manipulating stem cells in the right way, biomedical researchers can use them as a sort of "universal building material," cultivating just about any tissue or spare part needed.

At a company called Osiris Therapeutics in Baltimore, scientists extracted stem cells from goat's bone marrow and allowed them to multiply in a glass dish. Then they injected

10 million of these cells into the arthritic knees of goats. The tissues that had worn away began to grow back. The new growth from the stem cells also slowed the rate of continuing erosion, meaning stem-cell therapy holds the promise of prevention as well as repair. This would be true disease modification, rather than our current approach of just treating symptoms.

The same principle applies to the therapeutic use of a naturally occurring substance called bone morphogenetic proteins (BMP), which are produced on various occasions throughout our lives. They "turn on" for the first time before birth, when they spur growth in the fetus. After birth, these proteins "turn on" whenever we break a bone. Most tissues, when injured or cut, heal with a scar, which is different from what was there before. The healing tissue in bone, however, largely because of the action of BMPs, is identical to what was there before.

Scientists have now developed a genetically engineered form of BMP that's been approved by the U.S. Food and Drug Administration. These proteins induce bone formation and enhance fracture repair and can be used as an alternative for bone grafts in healing difficult fractures as well as in spinal fusion surgery, where solid healing is often a challenge. This means you don't have to "borrow" bone from somewhere else in the body. It basically comes in a jar off the shelf. You use it to induce the injured area to regenerate.

Bone is the only tissue that undergoes constant remodeling throughout life, retaining the capability to regenerate fully throughout adulthood. However, there are a variety of BMPs in our body, each with its own capacity to regenerate specific cells and tissue, not just bone. We're just beginning to learn of the potential impact of BMPs on tendons and on the articular cartilage that comprises your joint surfaces. Investigators in the musculoskeletal division of Wyeth Pharmaceuticals are working diligently to make these BMPs available clinically, both in the office and in the OR. The impact will be tremendous, with wide applicability in the treatment of a variety of musculoskeletal ailments.

These new technologies—BMPs, cell therapies, growth factors, and genetic engineering—are all geared to providing a quicker and more complete healing response. Whereas your body's natural ability may be limited in restoring normal form and function after injury, these promising interventions remove the biological barriers and limits to repair and regeneration.

KNEE POTHOLES AND THE ROAD CREW

Some knee injuries create "potholes" on the knee joint's protective cushion or cartilage, leaving areas of exposed bone destined to become arthritic without serious intervention. Until recently, an orthopaedic surgeon's best way to repair these articular cartilage potholes was to drill or "microfracture" the crater in order to create scar tissue to fill the cavity. This repair tissue is not very durable, and the results are usually temporary, often doing little to prevent the onslaught of arthritis.

But now specialists have an alternative way to "resurface" damaged knee cartilage. The procedure is called autologous chondrocyte implantation, or ACI. Healthy cartilage cells—

the chondrocytes—are harvested from the patient during a simple arthroscopic procedure, grown in a culture, then reimplanted in the damaged area, where they grow into healthy new cartilage tissue. The cells, more than 12 million new chondrocytes, are in a liquid suspension no larger than a thimble. They'll spill out of the defect if you just squirt them in, so the surgeon steals a bit of periosteum, the fibrous membrane that covers bones from the shinbone, to use as a patch to hold the new cells in the hole. Then the patch is carefully sutured to the joint surface (like a blowout patch on a tire) and sealed with an adhesive. Reports show ACI to be highly successful, with nearly 9 in 10 patients experiencing good results. I've performed many of these innovative procedures and have been very impressed with the results my patients have experienced. Their knees are actually getting a second chance. Focal areas of joint surface damage (i.e., "potholes"), including large areas, can be restored to a near normal condition.

Surgeons in Europe have taken ACI to the next level by impregnating the cultured chondrocytes into a bioabsorbable collagen scaffold or patch that can be implanted into the knee through smaller incisions, in a less invasive manner, with quicker recovery for the patient. This Matrix-Induced Autologous Chondrocyte Transplantation, or MACI, once available in the United States, will promote wider use of this knee saving technology.

What we can't do yet is repair the road, something that would be needed to restore larger areas of arthritic joint surface wear and damage. I believe this is coming soon with expanded use of chondrocyte transplantation in conjunction with other cell therapies. You can learn more about ACI by visiting www.carticel.com and www.matrixaci.com.

SCAFFOLDS FOR YOUR FRAME

Often, regeneration requires a scaffold to support the new growth. To make rotator cuff and ACL repairs, surgeons use a product from pig's intestines, a layer of cells called the submucosa. They sew the pig tissue patch into the torn tendon, and over time, the body creates new tissue around the area, with the body absorbing the remaining pig tissue. About 1,000 of these scaffolds have been implanted by U.S. doctors.

The same idea applies to meniscus transplants, where the surgeon makes a scaffold out of purified bovine collagen and puts it into the knee. This is important especially in a younger athlete or active individual who has a badly torn, unrepairable meniscus in the knee. Removing that important shock absorber can easily lead to premature arthritis. For this reason, whenever possible, we repair rather than remove a torn meniscus, or replace it with a donor meniscal allograft. Because of advances in polymer science and biomaterials, there is now the possibility of having reabsorbable polymer scaffolds, similar to the sutures used in current operations. The polymer scaffold is absorbed and disappears as the new tissue regenerates.

The logical extension of regenerative medicine is the actual genetic reprogramming of cells. Cynthia Kenyon, PhD, a researcher at the University of California at San Francisco, has doubled the life span of worms just by altering a single gene called daf-2. Kenyon's worms live six times as long as normal, the equivalent of 500 human years. What's more, the super-old worms look and act young. The daf-2 gene makes a protein similar to the human insulin receptor. Scientists suspect that it may respond to environmental signals—the smell of other animals, for instance, indicating overcrowding—to regulate life span. Whether or not this theory is accurate, the genetically modified Methuselah worms add credence to the idea that aging is a programmed biological function and not just the inevitable result of simple wear and tear. But no matter how long it takes scientists to solve the problem of programmed aging in humans, and I suspect it will take awhile, it's up to us to do what we can to manage the wear and tear part. That's what the mindful exercise and nutrition of the FrameWork program is all about. Researchers are helping the cause with cutting-edge techniques that ease pain and promote healing. Some of these are quite simple and involve merely finding new purposes for familiar medicines.

BOTOX FOR YOUR BOD AND SHOCKING SOLUTIONS

Botulinum toxin type A, for instance, now familiar as the temporary wrinkle-fix Botox—has long been used to treat uncontrolled muscle spasms in cerebral palsy, as well as chronic eye-muscle spasms. The toxin prevents nerve cells from releasing a chemical that triggers muscle contractions, which stops the spasms.

Aside from relaxing and lengthening chronically contracted muscles, Botox may also block certain pain-promoting proteins in the body, thus dampening any signals sent to the central nervous system.

Studies show that Botox injections may help ease stubborn pain in the neck and upper back when other treatments fail. In the studies, a single round of Botox injections coupled with physical therapy brought pain relief within a month. These studies are very preliminary and involve Botox only for reducing muscle spasms and controlling pain. If there really were a true Botox equivalent for muscles and tendons, an injection that could turn back the clock for those tissues the way Botox currently works for skin, it would be an overnight multibillion dollar product.

Another cutting-edge approach to pain is a technique called lithotripsy that uses a spark plug to generate shock waves to disrupt scar tissue. By causing microscopic damage to that tissue, the shock waves induce new blood vessel formation in the injured area and facilitate the healing process. They address the limiting factor in much problematic tissue healing: circulation, especially microcirculation. First used to noninvasively break up and treat kidney stones, this technology is now being applied to chronic tendinitis (tennis elbow, golfer's elbow, jumper's knee) as well as chronic heel pain (heel spurs, plantar fasciitis). Any chronically inflamed tendon is fair game.

SOUND HEALING

The exact mechanism by which ultrasound helps fractures heal is not known, but because bones grow in response to being physically stressed, the accelerated healing may be the result of the intense mechanical pressure that its pulsing waves deliver. The Sonic Accelerated Fracture Healing System (Exogen) is a hand-held, battery-operated device that delivers ultrasound pulses directly through the skin or through a small hole in a cast if necessary. Professional athletes and dancers, for whom every day counts in terms of healing, can now use this device at home when dealing with broken bones and even stress fractures.

Coblation microtenotomy uses radio waves to promote the growth of blood vessels in and around damaged tendons. This minimally invasive surgical procedure uses the Topaz device (a small, hand-held wand) to repair areas of tendon damage and avoid larger surgical procedures. High voltage, usually between 100 and 300 volts, combined with an electrically conductive fluid (usually isotonic saline), creates an ionized vapor layer, or plasma, of charged particles to transmit energy to the affected area, encouraging repair and remodeling of the damaged tissue.

LUBE JOB FOR YOUR JOINTS

For osteoarthritic pain in the knee, surgeons use synthetic lubricants to restore the lost joint-cushioning properties of synovial fluid. Synovial fluid produced in joints with osteoarthritis (OA) is thinner and thus less effective in its lubrication and shock-absorption capabilities. One of the reasons for the thinning of the liquid is the loss of hyaluronic acid. Doctors introduce Synvisc, an injectable form of hyaluronic acid directly into the knee, where it can relieve pain and improve function for up to 6 months (sometimes longer in my experience) by acting as a lubricant. Viscosupplementation (VS) or joint fluid therapy, as

this is called, does a good job of relieving arthritic knee pain and has a longer duration of relief than steroid or cortisone injections, all without the unwanted cortisone side effects.

Synvisc is a high-molecular-weight version of hyaluronic acid obtained in part from the comb of a rooster (i.e., chicken soup for your knee). It's FDA approved for use in knee osteoarthritis (OA), although orthopaedic surgeons use it in a variety of joints with OA, including the hip, elbow, ankle, and small joints of the hands and feet. Treatment involves three simple injections done in the office one week apart. Relief comes usually within 1 to 6 weeks.

Researchers have reported on the effectiveness of Synvisc in treating shoulder rotator cuff tendinitis and impingement syndrome, a tendon-related problem. Furthermore, studies are being done using VS for arthritis in other joints such as the hip.

I use the post-Synvisc improvement that my patient's experience to get them to do more things for themselves (exercise and weight loss) that will give a more lasting relief as the Synvisc wears off. It works across all grades or degrees of arthritis, from early damage to severe "bone on bone" situations, although it is much more effective in the earlier phases. It can be used for repeat treatment as well. With so many younger individuals experiencing knee osteoarthritis, viscosupplementation can help buy time until a joint replacement is needed or until many of the promising innovations for joint restoration and renewal become a reality. You can learn more about this "chicken soup" at www. synvisc.com.

COMPACT DISKS

For degeneration in the lower back, the latest solution is a prosthetic disk. Disks are made of firm cartilage on the outside with a pulpy middle. When the pulpy middle becomes brittle, damaged, or herniated, the pain can be constant and crippling. Until recently, spinal fusion was the method of choice for ending the pain, but relief came at a price. Removing the damaged disk and fusing the vertebrae together disrupts the mechanics of the entire back. Nearby vertebrae get more than their share of stress, and that can mean more pain. But now, a polyethylene, steel-plated prosthesis is available. Surgeons go in from the front of the body using small puncture holes in the abdomen so they won't have to move spinal nerves or touch the spinal cord as they take out the bad disk and replace it with the synthetic one. Two hours later, patients are up and walking. After 6 weeks, there are no physical restrictions (compared with 4 months for spinal fusion). Other countries have been using disk prostheses for more than a decade with superb results, but the procedure is still in the final experimental stages in the United States. Researchers have also developed prosthetic disks for the neck area, but these cervical disk replacements remain experimental.

IMAGE COUNTS

Improved diagnostic tools also are being brought into the effort to anticipate and head off musculoskeletal problems. Traditional imaging, such as MRI and x-ray, does not necessarily show accumulated wear and tear until it is well advanced. Newer, high resolution 3-D type MRI and bone scan imaging technology, however, now give doctors a chance to see the joint at the metabolic level.

Biomarkers obtained through a blood test may also allow us to predict and prevent joint wear. During the process of degradation that leads to osteoarthritis, molecules of connective tissue matrices are released into biological fluid. Researchers in France and Denmark have identified these molecules as markers for type II collagen and synovial tissue destruction. This allows doctors to identify patients who are most likely to face a rapid onslaught of arthritis while there is still time to prevent overt degenerative changes.

THE NOT-SO DEEPEST CUT

Even the surgical treatments that have been available for years have gotten much better because of technological research and advancement. These include better screws, plates, and rods for fractures, and now even bioabsorbable screws to hold ligaments in place while they are becoming part of your body, and bioabsorbable tacks to repair, rather than remove, torn menisci in the knee and torn labrum in the shoulder.

Most procedures are now being done on an outpatient basis via arthroscopy through tiny puncture holes or arthroscopic-assisted with "mini-open" incisions. Spine surgery is done "keyhole," with microscopic magnification so one can tread delicately around important neural structures. Minimal incision surgery, or MIS, is the rage, even for hip and knee replacements, which are lasting longer because of improved designs and techniques.

As I have said before, our first goal, even as surgeons, should be prevention. We are spending more than one trillion dollars on healthcare in the United States and only about 2 percent goes to prevention. The rest is spent on patchwork after things go wrong. We will never solve out-of-control healthcare costs until our focus shifts from being Dr. Fix-Its to prevention doctors. New treatment technologies are wonderful, but they're expensive, and the costs keep going up. The much better value for dollars comes from investing in prevention, which is where you reap the truly big dividends.

A NEW ERA

Worldwide, research on bone and joint health is accelerating, with the promise of good things to come. In fact, 2002 to 2011 has been designated by the United States and other nations as the "bone and joint decade." (See www.usbjd.org for more information.) Officially launched at the World Health Organization headquarters in Geneva, Switzerland, the International Bone and Joint Decade has been endorsed by nearly 40 nations, by all 50 U.S. states, and by more than 750 organizations worldwide. Goals of the decade include advancing research in prevention, diagnosis, and treatment of musculoskeletal disorders.

With remarkable advances just around the corner, there's never been a greater incentive to hang on to what you have through proper exercise, nutrition, and some simple lifestyle changes.

FIT FOR WHAT?

WITH THE FRAMEWORK PLAN, you will look better, feel better, and have a more durable frame that should last a lifetime. But exercise and fitness should never be an end unto itself.

The real purpose of improving your fitness is so you can enjoy an active life more fully. That goal extends far beyond any gym or workout. Being active then returns the favor by enhancing your overall fitness.

I've always loved sports. I started early with baseball, basketball, football, and even skateboarding. I then took up tennis and skiing after college and got pretty good. Later still, I advanced pretty far in the martial arts.

Most of these activities tapered off as I became busier as a surgeon. Now, because of time constraints, the only thing left is my workouts in the gym, which isn't good.

Looking back, I realize how each activity offered me a great deal in terms of improving my overall neuromuscular function, as well as my frame. I've remained fit, but I never fully realized the subtle loss of 3-D neuromuscular function—like balance and hand-eye coordination—until my children got me back into

skateboarding, ice skating, and tennis. Now I know what people mean when they say that kids will keep you young. The dropoff in my motor skills had been dramatic, but I hadn't noticed. These same motor skills are important in everyday life, not just in sports.

From a neurophysiological and biomechanical standpoint, there is only so much a one- or two-dimensional workout can give you. And "use it or lose it" applies to more than just muscle and bone.

For me, regaining these functions came back pretty easily, but I never would have regained them if I'd kept limiting myself to the gym.

So no matter how great you look or how terrific your workout or personal trainer is, find ways to put your health and fitness to good use with activities you enjoy. Remember, too, that it's never too late to take up new ones. Not everyone can do everything, but experiment to see what you like and what your frame can tolerate.

It's also never too early. Playing games with my children is not about me trying to relive my youth or fulfill some sports dreams. Rather it's an effort to instill in them lifetime habits of fitness and activity.

Our nation's children are more and more sedentary. Childhood obesity is an epidemic, and the best predictor of whether a child is active or a coach potato is the activity levels of their parents. If both parents are active, the child is five times more likely to be active than one of their friends with sedentary parents. If Dad alone is active, the child is three times more likely to be more active. Mom alone, two times. Clearly fitness needs to be a family activity.

I was at a function not long ago where Martina Navratilova, one of the fittest athletes on the planet, was asked about her off-court conditioning. She surprised everyone when she answered, "I play basketball (two-on-two full-court), soccer, ice hockey, and a variety of other activities. It all helps my game." Jet Li, martial arts master and action hero, uses badminton to improve his speed, focus, and explosiveness.

Today's focus on pushing kids into one particular sport early on is usually not a good idea. Playing soccer will help my kids become better tennis players, and playing tennis will make them better center fielders, and so on. Cal Ripken credits his baseball success on playing three sports in high school. "I think athleticism is developed by everything you do," he tells us. This explains why he tells his son, Ryan, to "put down your glove" when his baseball season is over.

Just as we can learn to read or speak a foreign language more easily at a certain age, we're also more receptive to neuromuscular programming when we're young. Also, neuromuscular pathways are wired early with regard to balance, proprioception, and hand-eye coordination. Starting early with a variety of activities wires kids for future skills. Some call it muscle memory, and it often comes back later if you need it.

Then again, it's better to start late than never get into the game. Your body was made to move. Thomas Cureton, an exercise physiologist, wisely noted that "the human body is the only machine that breaks down when not used." He's absolutely right.

We're living longer, and the FrameWork Program will help you live stronger and better for the whole ride. My hope is that it will allow you to do more than you've done before—in sports and in life—with comfort and ease.

TROUBLESHOOTING: THE ORTHOPAEDICS TOP 20 AND THEIR WORKOUT FIXES

WHILE WINDSPRINTS CAN BE GREAT training for an athlete, one mad dash can lead to hospitalization, or even sudden death, for someone with a heart problem.

Almost everyone seems to accept that distinction, but somehow the same cautionary logic hasn't extended to muscle-building exercises. Some strength-training exercises, while great for healthy young people, are dangerous for others. There may be nothing wrong with the routines themselves; they just aren't right for certain frames, especially when there is an overt or underlying musculoskeletal problem, i.e., a weak link.

This is why a vital part of the FrameWork Program is this collection of exercises modified for certain ailments. This slight adjustment in approach not only makes the movements safe, but also contributes to the repair and recovery of that weak link.

If you want to stay healthy, avoiding exercise is simply not an option.

So if you discover a problem—on the self-test (Step 1) or otherwise—it's no excuse for hanging up your workout clothes. You simply need to incorporate the appropriate modifications.

If you're under the care of a physician or therapist, especially if you've had recent surgery, it's always a great idea to run any exercises by him or her for approval.

THE TOP 20

Here are the most common ailments and injuries that orthopaedists see day in and day out, the ones that FrameWork aims to prevent. For more detailed information about these conditions, see the Sports Medicine section of my Web site, www.drnick.com, or the patient education area of the American Academy of Orthopaedic Surgeons (AAOS) Web site, "Your Orthopaedic Connection," at www.orthoinfo.aaos.org. Also, "The Body Almanac," published by AAOS is a good source of information on many common orthopaedic ailments. The exercise modifications and additions following each description should be included in your workout and/or rehabilitation. Remember, rehab-type exercises can and should be done daily, even several times a day until normal strength and/or flexibility are regained and you're feeling good. You often need several sets, especially a warmup with lighter weights or resistance for the strength exercises.

It's even more important to listen to your body, monitoring yourself for any significant discomfort or other changes to suggest you are getting further into trouble rather than out of it. This is especially true as you start to resume more normal workouts, although I recommend always giving your weak links a little added attention. As you expand your routine, especially as it involves the problem area or areas, don't add more than one new exercise per workout. While you're at the gym you often feel great, only to be sore or even in pain that evening or the following day. When you add more than one exercise, it's hard to know which is the culprit and needs either further modification or exclusion. You need to become a bit of a detective, monitoring things closely. And again, remember, if you're under the care of a physician or other health-care professional, always check with him or her about any changes in your program.

■ **All exercises mentioned in the Top 20 ailments "FrameWork Fix" area can be found in Step 3 (Core Connection) and Step 4 (Powerful Pliable Limbs), or in this section. By making the FrameWork program part of your everyday life, you can avoid these all-too-common ailments.**

ROTATOR CUFF PROBLEMS

From tendinitis to tears, this thin group of four strap muscles in the shoulder is the number one problem area for people who lift weights. It's also a huge problem for swimmers, even young ones, tennis and volleyball players, and baseball pitchers—anyone with repetitive, overhead activity.

The cuff rests between the collarbone and the acromioclavicular (AC) joint above, with the shoulder joint—the ball and socket—below. The peculiar location is why, with overhead use, the cuff gets pinched between this rock and a hard place.

Rotator cuff impingement leads to tendinitis. The cuff gets inflamed and starts to fray like a rope going back and forth over a cliff. It elongates, and then it tears.

Most exertion and fitness routines favor the front of the deltoid and the biceps at the expense of the rear deltoid and the rear part of the rotator cuff, creating muscle imbalance, which increases the likelihood of impingement. Creating balance in your workout to strengthen the rear cuff, as well as greater balance in your recreation activities, can guard against this scourge of the overhead slam.

■ **THE FRAMEWORK FIX:** Eliminate overhead lifts, especially barbell military press, behind-neck barbell press, and even dumbbell military press. Add Bow and Arrow (see page 111) and Internal and External Rotation rotator cuff exercises with elastic (see page 210). Modify side raises to unilateral (supported) and limit arc to painfree range. Do side raise variations "supraspinatus" (Empty Can) strengthening (see page 211). Add rear cuff lateral raise. Do rotator cuff stretches like the Pillar stretch, Arm cross stretch, Doorjamb stretch and TriSho stretch.

As your shoulder improves, you can gradually begin to introduce other lifts but remember, you may be prone to develop this again. When resuming overhead lifts, first try the dumbbell military press with very light weights (these are often better tolerated by those with shoulder ailments than the barbell versions). If symptoms return, cut back to the above program.

You can have huge deltoids and a weak rotator cuff. Do these rotator cuff specific exercises (both strength and stretching) regularly to keep your shoulders healthy and trouble free.

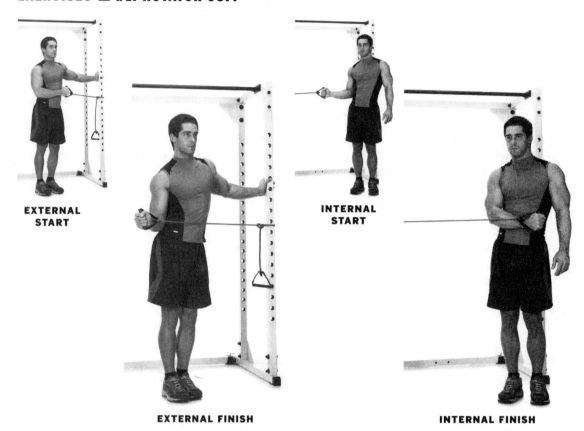

**EXTERNAL
START**

EXTERNAL FINISH

**INTERNAL
START**

INTERNAL FINISH

External Rotation (ER)/Internal Rotation (IR)

Fasten elastic tubing to a doorknob or other stationary object. Lock your right elbow to your side and do not lift off during exercises. To assure proper form, place a piece of paper or small towel between your elbow and your side the first few times you do this exercise; if the paper or towel drops, you're cheating. With your elbow flexed to 90 degrees and your elbow locked in, slowly rotate your arm outward, or external rotation, fully, pausing momentarily in the fully rotated position. Do 15 reps and then using the same arm perform internal rotation in which the arm is rotated inward against resistance. These exercises can also be performed using dumbbells while side-lying on a weight bench.

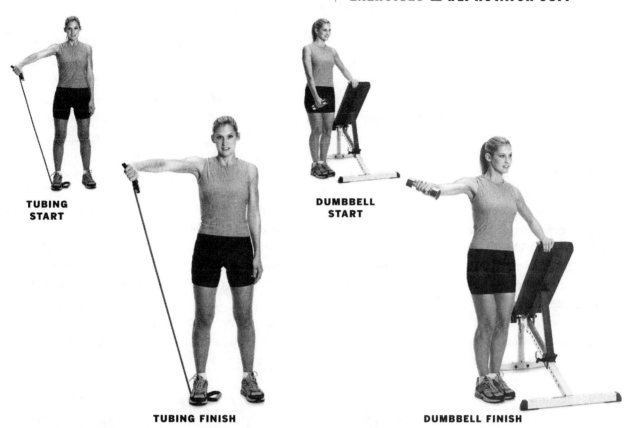

TUBING
START

TUBING FINISH

DUMBBELL
START

DUMBBELL FINISH

Supraspinatus ("Empty Can")

To isolate and strengthen the important supraspinatus rotator muscle, start with the elastic tubing. Stand on the tubing with your right leg, leaving enough slack to be able to pull the tubing from your waist area easily to your right shoulder. Hold the tubing thumbs down (as if you were emptying a can) with your entire arm forward approximately 30 degrees. Gently and slowly lift your arm (keeping thumb pointing down) until your hand comes up almost but not fully to shoulder height. Do 15 reps. This exercise can also be done with a very slight (i.e., 1 or 2 pounds) dumbbell. When the little but very important supraspinatus muscle is isolated, it doesn't take much weight or resistance to strengthen it or strain it, so start light and progress slowly.

"Tennis elbow" is tendinitis on the outer (lateral) side; "golfer's elbow" is tendinitis on the inside (the medial side). The inflammation can come from repetitive strain of any kind—from gardening, using a computer, and even operating a cash register.

The trouble arises from the number of powerful muscles for your fingers, hands, and forearms that all attach at one spot. On the palm side, you have all the flexing and pronating muscles attached to the inner side of your elbow. On the lateral side, you have finger, wrist, and forearm extensors, as well as the supinators (the muscles that let you rotate your palm upward like a bowl). The whole system is prone to overload, and familiar exercises such as negative chipups can attack that weak link at the elbow. Faulty technique is often the culprit. For golfers, cutting too deeply and whacking the turf is the prime culprit. For tennis players, it can be that the racket handle is too big or too small, or that you're hitting your backhand improperly or too late. Sometimes an hour or two with a coach or teaching pro can prevent hours with an orthopaedist or physical therapist.

■ *THE FRAMEWORK FIX:* Add forearm stretches including the Policeman's Stop forearm stretch and the Greedy Maitre d' (see below). Do forearm massage and wrist and forearm strengthening with elastic or dumbbell. Do four-way (not just extension and flexion but also wrist abduction and adduction). Finger wiggles or wave with wrist fully flexed and also fully extended.

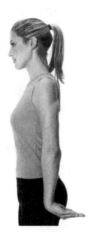 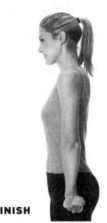

START   FINISH

Greedy Maitre d'

For forearm extension and flexibility, start with your arm at your side, wrist fully flexed to 90 degrees with fingers pointing behind you, palm facing upward. Keeping your wrist fully flexed, rotate your arm and hand around as far as it will go so your fingers are now pointing outward, away from you. Hold 5 seconds and repeat twice.

REPETITIVE STRAINS SUCH AS CARPAL TUNNEL SYNDROME

In 2000, carpal tunnel syndrome was the single leading cause of days missed from work. The carpal canal is a passage through the wrist containing one nerve and many different tendons. When the tendons are overworked, as from typing or from repetitive grasping in weight training, the nerve can become compressed or irritated. In the past, surgery was usually the remedy of choice, but now we more often recommend stretching exercises, massage, and even yoga.

■ **THE FRAMEWORK FIX:** Eliminate lifts that require heavy grasping by modifying exercise machines or use tubing. Add hand and forearm stretches and forearm massage. Take frequent breaks from computer work (keyboard and mouse) and stretch numerous times during the day. Correct your workstation (i.e., ergonomic redesign to protect you). Do both forearm stretches with elbows straight and then "prayer hands"; reverse prayer hands with elbows bent. These exercises help mobilize the involved nerve and are similar to "nerve glide" maneuvers done in therapy. Also include TriSho Stretch.

For ulnar neuritis (pinched nerve at elbow resulting in numbness in the small and ring finger innervated by the ulnar nerve and possible weakness of grip strength). Fully flexing the arm (especially suddenly) can stretch and irritate the ulnar nerve as it winds around the inner side of your elbow. Traditional biceps curls can irritate things, so try either not fully flexing your elbow upward during the lift or try Hammer Curls: Instead of supinating the forearm and having palms up at the end of the lift, keep palms facing inward throughout the full lift up and down. Add the above "nerve glide" stretches. Also, ulnar neuritis often accompanies golfer's elbow (or medial epicondylitis), so perform the exercises listed on the opposite page if tendinitis is part of the problem.

KNEE JOINT ARTHRITIS AND HIP JOINT ARTHRITIS

When the articular cartilage that cushions the joint surface wears out, you have arthritis, the number one cause of disability and activity limitation in the United States. Exercise can be of huge benefit in arthritis, or great harm, depending on how it's done.

Much about arthritis is out of our control. Researchers have just discovered, for instance, that there is a specific gene for arthritis of the knee. Being knock-kneed (genu valgus) or bowlegged (genu varus) makes arthritis more likely, as does prior injury and certain activities. A contributing factor we can do something about is obesity. Carrying around too much weight puts an undue strain on hips and knees—creating and accelerating arthritic wear.

In the old days before arthroscopic surgery, injury meant removing the entire meniscus through major open surgery, which invited arthritis, which then led to a staggering number of knees being replaced. Now we're on the second round, replacing the replacements.

What follows are ways of ensuring that spare parts are not in your future. You need stretching, but stretching is about muscle; it's range-of-motion exercises that address the joints per se. A good workout includes both.

■ **THE FRAMEWORK FIX:** For knee joint arthritis, eliminate high impact exercises. Add bicycle, elliptical, or water exercises. Do quad isometrics (page 218); if tolerated, move up to "short arcs," then to leg extensions. Add quad and hamstring stretching. Do knee range-of-motion exercises (page 216) to gain or maintain mobility. Do calf strengthening.

For hip joint arthritis, eliminate high impact exercises. Add bicycle, elliptical, or water exercises. Do hip range-of-motion exercises (never force to regain range), including Knee-to-Chest stretch, Straddle stretch, T-Roll, and Pretzel stretch (see page 82). Strengthen hip with elastic or machines within your comfort range. Include Can Opener (see page 232). For strength include exercises for hip abductor, adductor, hip flexors, and gluteal area. Good water exercise is to hold a kickboard, noodle, or wear a buoyancy vest (AquaJogger or Wet Vest) and do a cross-country ski maneuver (scissors-type back and forth) with your legs (bending mostly at the hip but not at the knees). Many individuals with hip degenerative joint disease and limited hip mobility get lower back and sacro-iliac pain or dysfunction, so it is also wise to do lower back pain preventive exercises (see page 231–233).

The bursa is a thin layer of tissue that helps lubricate the tissues surrounding a joint. Inflammation of the bursa (bursitis) located at the hip is a problem more common in women than in men, perhaps because of the generally wider female pelvis. When muscles and tendons on the outer side of the hip rub on the bone prominence called the greater trochanters, it creates friction underneath. Exercising the outer thigh to increase strength and flexibility can offset the friction.

■ *THE FRAMEWORK FIX:* Check for discrepancy in leg length and compensate with orthotic or heel lift if one leg is longer than the other. Do Pretzel stretch (see page 82) and T-Roll (see page 83). Strengthen with elastic or machines, including Hip Abductor (most important) and Hip Adductor (see page 128), and gluteal exercises (i.e., Hamstring Kickback, below).

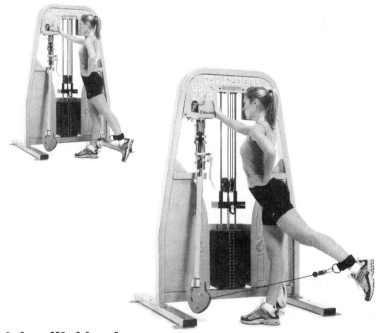

Hamstring Kickback

Do not arch the back. Do not throw weight rapidly.
Let weight back down slowly in a controlled manner.

KNEE CARTILAGE TEAR

Along with childbirth and hysterectomies, arthroscopic knee surgery is the most common hospital procedure in America, and it's usually performed for cartilage tears.

This injury is to baseball catchers what turned ankles are to basketball players. Football players tear cartilage when they're hit from behind or do a sudden twist. Weight lifters tear theirs by using poor form on deep squats—bouncing in sudden exertion when trying to lift too much weight. Plumbers, auto mechanics, and other "squatters" can get a rip just doing their jobs. So can mothers helping their kids "button up."

The meniscus—two "C"-shaped shock absorbers in each knee, one on the inner side and one on the outer side—simply dries out and weakens with age. When that happens, you can tear your cartilage just getting out of a car or working in your garden. Then you need arthroscopic surgery, which isn't so bad, but in removing the damaged cartilage, you are also removing a shock absorber. So that gives you another weak link. Stronger surrounding muscles can compensate to some extent. To protect your knees, give that surrounding tissue a good workout. Meanwhile, be mindful of other ways to both lower the stresses on your knees and improve the shock absorption.

■ **THE FRAMEWORK FIX:** Add stationary bicycling, which is great to build both quad strength and endurance to help with knee shock absorption. Do quad strengthening, knee range-of-motion exercises, calf and hamstring strengthening, hip strengthening (abductor and adductor) and functional drills (see ACL Tear on page 220).

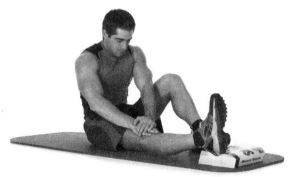

KNEE EXTENSION

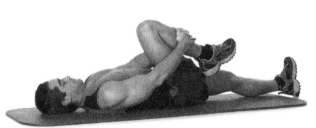

KNEE FLEXION

Knee Range of Motion

Place your heel on a phone book and gently press downward on your knee until it's fully extended. Hold for 5 seconds. Next, flex your knee and gently pull your heel toward your buttocks.

PATELLAR PAIN SYNDROME

An irritated patella (kneecap) is the number one knee problem among younger people. During adolescence, growth spurts in bones sometimes mean that muscle and tendons can't keep up, which leaves kids with dangerously tight hamstrings. Malalignment can mean that the kneecap doesn't ride properly in its groove. In adults, the same condition is created by overuse and imbalance—as in too much running without adequate stretching and strengthening exercises to offset the self-imposed imbalances and tightness.

With age and with injuries, simple wear and tear leads to degenerative arthritis under the kneecap. Most exercises that strengthen the thigh will irritate this already troubled spot, so you have to be very smart and strategic in your workouts. In this context, step aerobics, squats, and leg extensions are all "X-rated," meaning that you don't go there. Quadriceps strengthening is the an-

swer, but it has to be done so as not to overload the kneecap. Hamstring and iliotibial band (ITB) stretching are also essential.

■ *THE FRAMEWORK FIX:* Eliminate usual quad exercises (leg extensions, lunges, squats). Add "lock and lift" isometrics (see page 218); or "lock out" or "pin out" the weight stack on machines. If tolerated, then go to "Short Arc" isotonics (concentration VMO) and T-Band Pumps (see page 122). Stretch hamstrings, quads, and the ITB. Also strengthen hip adductors (most important) and hip abductors. Add stationary bicycle but with a higher seat, no hills, and use toe clips, or use the elliptical. Avoid stairsteppers, especially many of the inexpensive home versions that might not be as smooth for your knee. If you are using a stepper, keep the step action on one of the lower settings. Consider a knee sleeve (neoprene with an open patella).

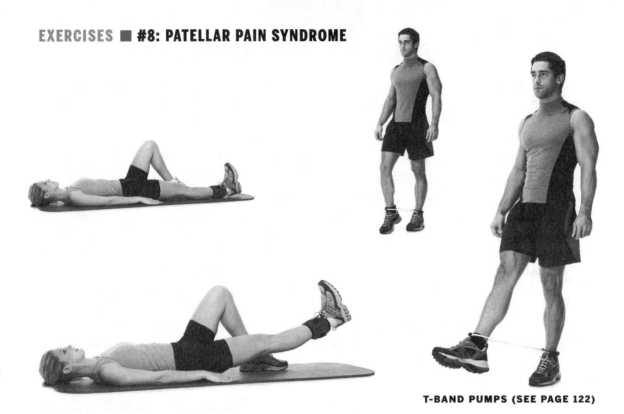

T-BAND PUMPS (SEE PAGE 122)

"Lock-and-lift" isometrics

These are for quad strength, especially for individuals with patellar pain syndrome or patello-femoral arthritis, or anyone in the early phases of knee rehabilitation, especially post-op, including arthroscopy. All too often I see motivated individuals rehabbing their knees, trying to strengthen their quad muscles when their "cheatin' bod" is playing tricks. This is especially true when you are doing quad isometrics, or straight leg lifts, when your body is wrongly using your hip flexors, not your quadriceps and especially not your important VMO portion of the quad, to raise the leg.

To avoid this, I developed the concentration "lock-and-lift" exercise.

Lie on your back with your left knee bent and left foot resting on the ground. Next tighten and slowly lock your right thigh (pushing back with the right knee). Feel the VMO muscle (teardrop-shaped muscle on the inner side of the knee just above the kneecap). Be sure it contracts and gets firm. Next lift your right leg 6 to 8 inches off the ground and hold 5 to 7 seconds. Keep feeling your thigh muscle and VMO to be sure they are staying tight at maximal contraction (until you get really good at this). Hold 5 to 7 seconds and repeat 12 to 15 times. When this gets very easy, start adding ankle weights (start with 1 to 2 pounds and don't go over 10 pounds, or you will probably start using your hip again to do the lift). The key is concentrating on tightening and palpating the muscle for biofeedback-type information to assure you are really working the muscle effectively.

INFRAPATELLAR TENDINITIS (JUMPER'S KNEE)

This is an all too common complaint among basketball and volleyball players, as well as dancers, so much so that they often think it's normal to get a "pinch" of pain when they jump or land. Runners feel it, too, especially on a downhill slope. Usually, a tight, overdeveloped quadriceps muscle is putting a strain on the tendon that lives just below the kneecap. The answer is quad stretching, as well as exercises that emphasize the eccentric or lengthening contraction on the muscle, the one we experience when we properly (i.e., slowly) lower a weight.

■ *THE **FRAMEWORK** FIX:* Add transverse friction massage, quad, hamstring, and calf stretching and Eccentric Quad Strengthening (see below). Consider a "cho-pat" strap (a band that goes around the knee just below the tip of the kneecap) or a knee sleeve.

If you are a runner or walker, avoid hills or banked surfaces. For cycling, check your bike seat adjustment (up/down and front/back) and use toe clips. Also, be sure you are riding the correct frame size.

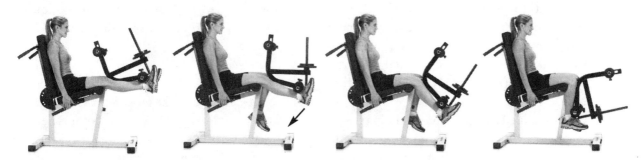

Eccentric Quad Strengthening

Do double leg extensions then relax uninvolved leg down and lower the weight with the involved side only. This allows for negative or eccentric quad work.

ACL TEAR (TRICK KNEE)

This is an injury that is its own epidemic, especially among women. A female athlete is four to five times more likely than a male to tear her ACL, the anterior cruciate ligament. This ropelike band of tissue runs right through the center of the knee and helps to hold the joint together. When it tears, the shin bone (tibia) can slide forward in relation to the thigh bone (femur). That's the "trick" in a trick knee, an excruciatingly painful stunt you'll never want to repeat.

This condition is so prevalent among active young women that I've treated as many as three players from the same field hockey team—in the same season—for ACL tears. But the one group that seems almost immune is dancers. In 20 years of working with these women, I've probably seen a total of four or five torn ACLs. What's the secret of these bionic ballerinas? Dancers are among the greatest athletes on the planet and in terms of preventing certain injuries, that conditioning pays off. And it's not just routine strength and flexibility that counts here. It's much more specific. I think it's their fine-tuned balance, coordination, and proprioception (your body's internal balance coordination mechanisms), as well as exceptionally well-balanced muscle training. More importantly, ballet dancers learn to jump and land properly, even as little kids. Early and continued jump training (especially the landing, which is more important in terms of ACL tear prevention) holds the key to their knee protection. Research has shown that females land differently than males, and that either a stiff-legged landing or more commonly a landing in which the knee buckles inward, even slightly (both happen more so in girls), predispose girls to ACL tears. Also, data suggests that boys and girls seem to jump and land pretty equally until their adolescent growth spurt, after which boys continue to improve in jumping and landing. It is around the time of maturation that the incidence of ACL tears rises dramatically in girls, who are four to six times more likely to tear their ACLs. Surgery can repair most of the damage, but prevention, by strengthening the hamstrings and quads and by improving proprioception, agility, and balance the way dancers do, is vastly preferable.

■ **THE FRAMEWORK FIX:** Take a lesson from the dancers who, unlike most female athletes, rarely ever tear their ACLs. Do comprehensive leg and knee strengthening, especially hamstrings. Backward walking on a treadmill helps recruit and strengthen hamstrings. Add Tai Chi moves, dance, balance exercises, and single-leg hopping for proprioception. Core strength is also protective.

If you have had ACL surgery, especially in the first 6 months post-op, you should follow your surgeon's guidelines for recovery. I believe in a fairly aggressive rehab program starting almost immediately post-op, but every surgeon is different depending on his or her philosophy, type of graft and techniques used, and method of graft fixation in the knee. If you are more than 6 months out of surgery, or if you are trying to live without an ACL (i.e., the ligament tore and you never had surgery), then the following routines will be helpful.

This **Wobble board, or the Bosu variant,** is a small platform that rests on a half ball. By practicing balancing and standing on this inherently unstable object, you can significantly improve your proprioception.

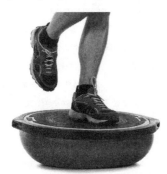

BOSU BALANCE TRAINER

Four-quadrant hopping drills. After you are able to comfortably hop in place (equally injured to uninjured side), skip rope, and/or shadow-box comfortably, this more advanced exercise can be helpful to your knee rehab effort. Jump one-legged bunny hops in four directions (front, back, and side to side). Compare right to left for deficits. As you get better, the hops can be higher and further in each direction.

Functional drills: There is only so much you can do in the gym, training room, or rehab setting to prepare your knee for full return to sports and other leisure activities. To prepare yourself for that final phase after any knee surgery or rehabilitation, you should work through a variety of functional progressions. In some instances, a knee brace is a good idea (check with your doctor). Once you are comfortable jogging straight ahead on a treadmill, and then on a smooth flat track surface, you can start some running and cutting drills on a field. These include running "flair-out" patterns like a football receiver going out for a pass. Jog forward in a straight line approximately 10 yards. Then, as you continue to jog, slightly angle off either to the right or left as if you were driving a car going off an exit ramp with a gentle curve. Start with gentle flairs at half speed going to the right and left and progress to faster speeds and sharper curves. You can also "stop on the dime" and do a 90-degree turnout both right and left. Also, jogging figure-eight patterns are very helpful. Start slowly over a 20-yard distance and gradually increase your speed and tighten the figure-eights to 10 yards.

We are now learning that many ACL tears are preventable with certain year-round conditioning programs, especially those that focus on strengthening and functional drills, including jumping and landing drills. These programs seem especially important to young female athletes who are tearing their ACLs at epidemic rates. I believe that every young athlete, especially females, should be on an ACL preventive program as part of their routine practices and training on and off the field. Programs like the Santa Monica ACL Prevention Project are excellent. You can find more information at www.aclprevent.com.

ITB FRICTION SYNDROME

The iliotibial band is a thick, tendonlike structure on the outer side of the knee, and repetitive movement there can create friction bursitis. Cyclists and runners get this frequently, and technical factors play a big role. For cyclists, it's not just the height of the seat that matters but its place forward or aft. The problem for runners is often banked surfaces or legs that are uneven in length.

■ *THE FRAMEWORK FIX:* Try the Pretzel stretch, ITB stretch (at right), and T-Roll. Consider orthotics. Check knee alignment and leg-length discrepancy. Do hip abductor and adductor strengthening with elastic (see page 128). If you are a runner or walker, avoid banked surfaces. If you bike, check your bike seat adjustment (up/down and front/back) and use toe clips.

ITB stretch. Lie on your left side with your legs straight. Using your right hand, pull your right foot back toward your right buttock and extend your right hip backward slightly. Next drop your right knee back and lower it toward the ground behind your left knee. Hold for 10 to 20 seconds and repeat twice.

The two most common pulls are of the hamstrings and the groin. The groin is the adductor or inner side muscle of the hip, the one that pulls one leg in toward the other. The hamstring is the big muscle in the back of the thigh. Calf strains are also very common, and just about any muscle in your body can tear. Trouble usually comes from sudden acceleration in running, but tight muscles are the underlying problem. When you strain a muscle it heals, but with scar tissue that's less elastic than the healthy tissue it replaced. The right kind of treatment—which is immediate treatment—can make a big difference in the kind of scar that forms. But again, prevention is even better. Stretching is the key to loosening up these muscles and making them behave, as well as strengthening exercises that emphasize the lengthening contraction or eccentric pressure. Proprioceptive neuromuscular facilitation (PNF) techniques are particularly helpful for tight-jointed individuals or those with recurrent muscle pulls.

■ **THE FRAMEWORK FIX:** Do area-specific strengthening and PNF stretching (see "PNF Stretching" on page 102) and eccentric workouts to prevent strain. Try massage, including transverse friction. Conduct longer periods of warmup and stretching, especially the involved muscle group. Remember warmup and stretching are different.

A neoprene sleeve can be helpful in keeping the involved area warm and less likely to strain. There are neoprene sleeves for almost every body area, including the upper thigh or groin, thigh, knee, and calf. Keep well hydrated and don't continue playing when fatigue sets in.

If you are in a stop-start sport, like baseball, be sure to warm up and stretch the involved area before starting up again, because your muscle-tendon complex can get quite cold and tight during the downtime.

This is a tear of the medial gastrocnemius, meaning the calf muscle on the inner side as it rises out of the Achilles tendon. You get the pull just about on the midpoint where your calf bulges. It most often happens when running, and the name is derived from the sharp pain that makes tennis players think they've been hit in the back of the leg with a ball. But it also happens to joggers and softball players, especially when making a stop-start movement. Tight calves are the culprit, along with dehydration, fatigue, and shoes with too-low heels.

■ *THE FRAMEWORK FIX:* Do calf stretching and strengthening (including "eccentric" on page 226). Progress to hopping drills and rope jumping. Avoid dehydration. Check height of heel in shoe. If you switch to a new brand with even a slightly lower heel, you can strain your calf area. If you still have slight tightness, consider using a temporary heel lift in your sneaker until you regain normal flexibility and strength.

A variety of muscles from the foot and ankle attach to the leg on the inner side of the shin. Repeated overload and overuse can strain this attachment. Shin splints aren't serious, but they need to be sorted out from stress fractures (see page 234), which are serious. Both dropped and high arches (pronated feet and flat feet) contribute to shin splints, as do improper shoes. But overdeveloped calves, relatively weak shins, and design flaws in your exercise program are the major causative factors. Stretching the calf, and using elastic to strengthen the shin, can bring the abnormal biomechanics under control.

■ *THE FRAMEWORK FIX:* Do calf stretching (see page 133) and Preacher Stretch (below). Use elastic exercises to strengthen shin, especially tibialis anterior (page 229) (front shin) but also ankle inversion/eversion (see page 228). Consider orthotics.

If you're a runner or walker, cut your mileage in half and if you are doing your program daily, make it every other day. Get a new pair of sneakers if yours are wearing down.

Be sure your shin pain is not a stress fracture or chronic exertional compartment syndrome (CECS); check with your sports medicine specialist. In addition to orthotics, a neoprene shin sleeve is sometimes helpful.

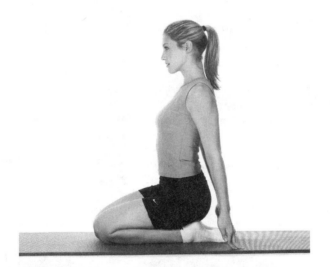

Preacher Stretch (Front Shin Stretch)

Sit back on your feet with your toes pointing directly backward. Hold for 10 to 20 seconds and repeat twice. If this is difficult for you because of discomfort in the knees or ankles, try a single foot version in which you are kneeling on the opposite knee. This allows you to let yourself back in a more controlled manner.

ACHILLES TENDINITIS

This is the number-one injury for runners, right alongside heel pain and plantar fasciitis (see page 230). With age, tendons begin to soften. The computerized image of an Achilles is usually jet black, but the MRIs of seasoned runners often show areas of white where the tendons are starting to fail. Part of the problem is overload, and part of it is imbalanced musculature from imbalanced workouts. Tight calves and tight heel cords are a setup for tendinitis, and repetitive overuse takes you the rest of the way. The answer, once again, is proper stretching and better balance in the workout to strengthen all the relevant muscles.

■ *THE FRAMEWORK FIX:* You should wait until the acute inflammation settles down (with RICE and meds) before starting these exercises. Do calf stretches (see page 133) and strengthening, including the Eccentric workout below and quad and shin strengthening. Progress to hopping exercises. If symptoms persist, consider an orthotic and a night splint (which actually keeps your Achilles comfortably on stretch all night rather than relaxed where it tightens up and hurts with the first steps in the morning.

Eccentric Calf workout. On a step, go up onto the balls of both feet, then lift off your uninvolved side so you are up on the ball of the foot of the involved side only. Slowly let yourself down until your heel drops way downward and you feel a good stretch in the Achilles or calf area. Hold for 5 seconds. Then using both feet, go back up. When you can easily do 20 reps, add weight by holding dumbbells in your hands.

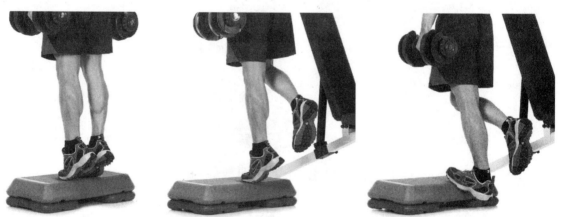

Eccentric Calf Workout

The number-one problem for basketball players, the number one acute injury for dancers, a common chronic condition among the general population, and a major nuisance for women who wear high heels is ankle sprains. To sprain an ankle means to stretch the ligament on the outer side, and once that happens, it's never quite as tight as before. Incomplete rehabilitation of the ankle (IRA) is a huge problem. Your ankle is still vulnerable because of subtle persistent weakness and tightness. Exercise will help get those ankles back in shape. You must also address proprioception, the fine-tuned coordination we lose very quickly any time there's injury and swelling to the lower extremity. Improved proprioception means your joint makes internal microsecond adjustments without your even knowing it to keep your ankle from giving way.

Primarily, you must make up for the laxity by strengthening certain little muscles, especially the peroneal muscles on the outer side of the ankle. As they get stronger, you are less likely to turn your ankle.

■ *THE FRAMEWORK FIX:* Do strengthening exercises when you're over the acute phase and the swelling and limp are getting better. Do Ankle Tubing exercises (below) for all muscles, especially the outer peroneal muscles. Do calf stretching (see page 133) and the Stork (see page 77) for proprioception, pillow stand for balance, and the wobble board. Consider an ankle support (figure-eight Velcro type) for activities to prevent recurrence.

Ankle Tubing exercises (see pages 228, 229). These are to strengthen peroneal muscles (ankle everters). Fasten a piece of elastic tubing under a sturdy chair leg. Wrap a loop around the forefoot area with mild tension on the band and your ankle relaxed slightly pointed downward. Using only ankle movement, not your leg, rotate your foot and ankle outward (like a windshield wiper) feeling the muscles on the outer side of your lower leg working. Pause for several seconds in the fully outward position and relax back slowly to the starting position. Do 15 to 20 reps. Next perform the same exercises only adjust the strap band so that you are pulling inward (ankle inverters). Finally place the band over the top of the foot so you are pulling your foot upward (ankle dorsiflexors) against resistance.

For recurrent ankle sprains, weak ankles, and ankle instability, the most important exercises include balance, peroneal strengthening, and calf stretching (a tight calf predisposes you to ankle sprains).

EXERCISES ■ #16: ANKLE SPRAINS

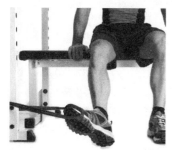

**ANKLE INVERSION
START**

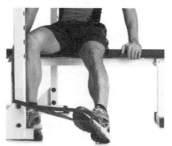

**ANKLE EVERSION
START**

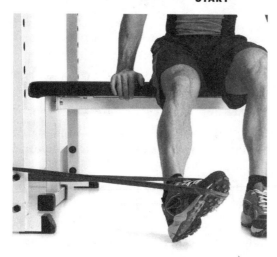

**ANKLE INVERSION
FINISH**

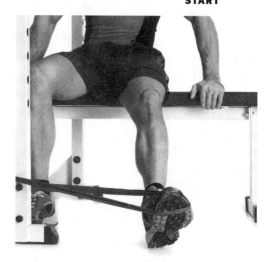

**ANKLE EVERSION (FOR PERONEALS)
FINISH**

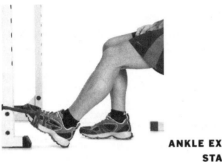

**ANKLE EXTENSION
START**

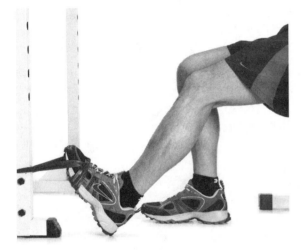

**ANKLE EXTENSION (FOR TIBIALIS ANTERIOR)
FINISH**

HEEL PAIN (PLANTAR FASCIITIS AND HEEL SPUR SYNDROME)

Heel pain can be the result of a bone spur or inflammation of the plantar fascia, the firm tendonlike band of tissue that attaches the muscles of the arch to the heel. Overuse and lack of shock absorption is the culprit, often made worse by a flat foot (pronated) or a foot with a high arch.

■ *THE FRAMEWORK FIX:* Do calf stretching (see page 133) and Arch (Plantar Fascia) Stretch (see below). Try arch massage with a golf or tennis ball. Do arch strengthening (put soup cans on a towel on the floor, pull toward you with your toes). Use a heel gel pad and a night splint. Orthotics can be helpful, but first try heel gel pads and over-the-counter inexpensive inserts before taking the plunge to an expensive custom orthotic. Stretching and a night splint are the key to this problem.

Repeat the Arch Stretch and barefoot calf stretching every few hours during the day. These are also good in the morning after massaging your arch, before even getting out of bed.

There are other possible causes of chronic heel pain besides plantar fasciitis or heel spurs. If pain persists, get it checked to assure no stress fracture, neurological, or rheumatologic problems.

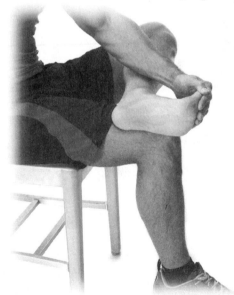

Arch (Plantar Fascia) Stretch

Sit with your shoe off. Cross your leg over the opposite knee so the involved foot is resting on the knee. Use your hand to pull or extend all your toes backward toward your shin while simultaneously bringing up your ankle. Hold for 10 to 20 seconds and repeat 2 to 3 times. You should feel a stretch in the arch area, even using your thumb to feel the tension on the arch area.

LOWER BACK PAIN (STRAIN, HERNIATED DISK, AND SCIATICA)

Backache was the price humans accepted when we adopted upright posture. We get to use our hands for carrying things instead of for walking, but 80 percent of the population at some time or another suffers a debilitating back strain. Unfortunately, it's not usually a one-time deal. Once invited in, backache tends to be a repeat visitor.

Along with the common cold, back strain is the number one reason people miss work, and the number one source of workers' compensation payments. Among 40 year olds, even those who've never had a back episode, MRI studies reveal that 30 percent show disk degeneration and sometimes even disk herniation. Tight hamstrings and weak hip flexors are also associated with low back trouble. Even smoking, which has a hugely negative impact on microcirculation, can contribute. Fitness and exercise protect against back attacks.

■ *THE FRAMEWORK FIX:* Conduct a full "back school" to refine bending and lifting techniques. Stretch hamstrings and lower back. Strengthen lower back, especially spinal extensors. Do Crunches (see page 84) to strengthen abs. Old-fashioned situps are definitely "X-rated." Use Pilates, Tai Chi, yoga, or other techniques (i.e., relaxation breathing) to lower stress and build core strength. Regular core work is essential. You should have a

Swiss Ball or Thera-Ball at home. Water exercise is ideal, especially if land or usual exercise is not tolerated. Remember cardio workouts are important not only to get the blood flowing and nourish your disks and other spinal support structures but also because improved aerobic capacity (i.e., better cardiovascular conditioning) has been shown scientifically to lower the incidence of lower back problems. Also it helps with weight control, another factor in lower back ailments. Again, water work is ideal, but walking, elliptical machines, and stationary cycling are also usually well tolerated. Avoid the rowing machine or outdoor biking where you are significantly flexed forward.

In addition to the above suggestions, add the following preventive exercises on pages 232 and 233 as tolerance allows.

If problems persist, find a gym or rehab center that has Med X lumbar rehabilitation and testing machines, which have helped countless lower back sufferers.

Also check your mattress. A significant amount of lower back discomfort is preventable with the right mattress. This is especially true for people who wake up with discomfort and morning stiffness in the spine. I like a mattress that is slightly firm but accommodating rather than a rigid plank design. See what works best for you. Many of my patients swear by the newer memory-foam designs.

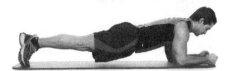

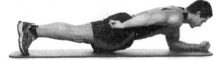

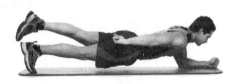

Quadriped

See description on page 56 in the self-test in Chapter 4.

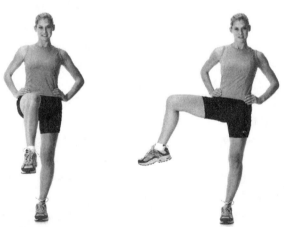

Standing "Can Opener"

Stand upright, flex right hip upward so it is at 90 degrees, approximately the height of your belt. Tighten your abs, performing an Ab-Hollow maneuver. Next keeping your abs tight and drawn in, slowly rotate your left leg and knee outward as far as it can go, then let your outwardly turned left foot downward to the ground so it forms a "T" with your right foot. Alternate sides, repeat each 3 to 5 times.

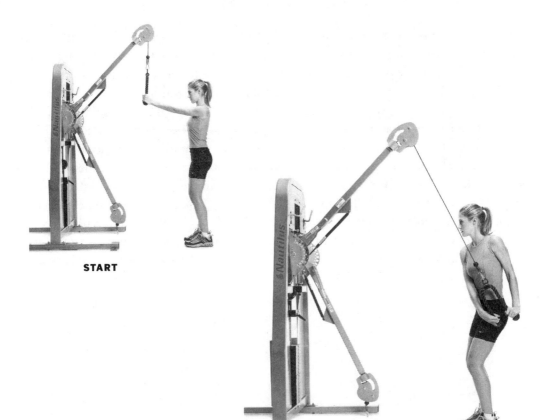

START

FINISH

"Twist-Os"

This is best done on a cable machine but can also be done with elastic tubing. Stand with your feet slightly wider than your shoulders. Hold the rope pulley with both hands in front of you and your arms out with elbows slightly bent. Tighten and hollow your abdominal area. Next, using your abdominal and torso area (not arms or lats) rotate your midsection and slowly bring your right hand down toward the outer side of your left thigh, pausing for a moment but keeping your abdominal area tucked in and tightened. Keep your shoulder and chest facing forward to better isolate and activate your abdominal core muscles. Return to the starting position and repeat to the opposite side. Do 5 to 7 reps on each side.

STRESS FRACTURES

Runners get stress fractures of the shin, but also at the hip. Dancers get them at the base of the second metatarsal bone in the foot, or on the outer side of the ankle. Gymnasts get stress fractures of the spine. Women who overtrain to the point of a dramatic loss in body fat suspend their usual flow of hormones, which leads to loss of bone density, which leads to a significantly higher incidence of stress fractures. More generally, stress fractures underscore the importance of exercise as a managed dose. Too much of a good thing can lead to damage.

■ *THE FRAMEWORK FIX:* Depending on the location, strengthen the surrounding musculature. Depending on the sports and fitness activity, work with a coach or trainer to redesign your program. Since so many overuse injuries, like stress fractures, are rooted in either faulty techniques or faulty program design, especially consider any sudden change or increase in intensity, duration, or frequency of the activity. For women, evaluate your menstrual cycle and improve the amount of calcium in your diet. For lower extremity stress fractures, consider orthotics.

NECK DEGENERATIVE DISEASE AND STRAINS

Like lower back pain, neck trouble can be the result of simple repetitive strain from typing on a computer or even just leaning over paperwork. Old sports injuries and auto accidents are also a huge factor in the prevalence of this condition. Football, even in teenagers, takes a heavy toll on the cervical spine. At the gym, too many of us do in our necks trying to go for that extra repetition on a shoulder press or a pulldown routine. All it takes is one sudden straining of the neck to create the weak link that then becomes a lifelong problem.

There is much you can do to avoid this kind of injury, as well as the simplest and most pervasive approach for most people in protecting the neck, which is to lower your general stress level. The same holds for the lower back, which is notorious for harboring and abetting stress. I can't send you off to Rancho Relaxo, but I can stress the importance of becoming more aware of how and where you carry stress in your body and the proper posture and alignment to offset that. You should also incorporate a few basic mind-body techniques, not only for your neck, but also to lower your potential for developing a stress-related condition anywhere in your musculoskeletal system.

■ **THE FRAMEWORK FIX:** Do range-of-motion (see page 75) and strengthening exercises (see page 236) for the neck. Add upper body strengthening but with lower weight and unilateral reps. Modify lifting technique to reduce neck compression forces. Do stress reduction including relaxation breathing and aerobic workouts. Walking and elliptical are ideal. Swimming can sometimes be problematic. If you are a swimmer, vary your stroke. If you are a cyclist, raise the handlebars. Handlebar extensions can be purchased at most bike shops. Also consider brake extensions so that if you are holding the upper center area of the handlebars, the brakes are within your grip rather than having to lean down to the usual hand grip/break area.

If problems persist, find a gym or rehab center that has MedX neck rehabilitation and testing machines that have helped countless neck sufferers.

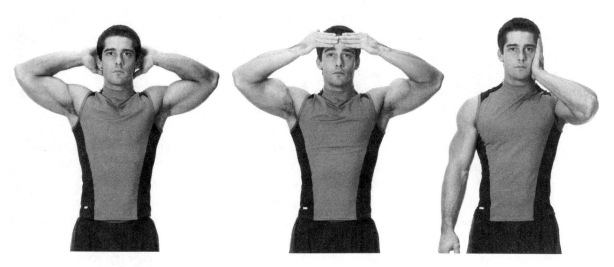

Neck Isometrics

Interlace your fingers and clasp your hands behind your head backward but resist the movement with your hands tightening your neck extensor (back of neck) muscles. Hold 5 to 7 seconds. Repeat 5 times. This type of isometric exercise should also be done by pressing against your forehead, and leaning your head forward as well as pressing on the right and left side of your head and leaning to each side. As an isotonic (moving) alternative, elastic tubing can be used in which a small amount of motion, rather than an isometric hold, can be added. This is done by placing the elastic band against your head for resistance. Keep the movement slow and within your painfree range. At the gym, seek out 4-way neck machines. Start with no weight and work in your painfree range.

BUILT TO LAST

If you've been lucky enough to avoid the Top 20 so far, congratulations. Unfortunately, time itself is causing changes in your body that make these far more likely to become your companions in the future. They are the bread and butter of orthopaedics, but the idea here is to make sure that you don't become toast.

If you have difficulty with these or other musculoskeletal ailments, get them checked out earlier rather than later. Often a simple rehabilitation program, like those offered nationwide at NovaCare Rehabilitation centers (www.novacare.com), can get you out of trouble. Better yet, put prevention to work now.

Monitor your body for signs and symptoms of these and other frame-related ailments. Also, perform the self-test regularly so you can nip things in the bud before they sideline you. The FrameWork Program should offer plenty of protection from these and most musculoskeletal problems. Follow the program every week, and you can count on being more durable for life, with a frame that's solid, a body that's built to last.

APPENDIX 2

■ ■ ■

SELF-TEST

EVERY SELF-TEST QUESTION has important implication for your frame (your musculoskeletal system). After reading *FrameWork* in its entirety, you will have a much clearer understanding of why most items were included. The following partial listing directs you to appropriate areas in the book for certain questions or topic—some general, some specific) from the self-test. For more detailed information, check out the interactive version of the *FrameWork* self-test at www.drnick.com.

■ Learn more about the Self-Test and what it means at www.drnick.com ■

■ ■ ■

■ Learn more about the Self-Test and what it means at www.drnick.com ■

INDEX

Boldface page references indicate photographs and charts. <u>Underlined</u> references indicate boxed text.

A

Abdominal strength self-test, 59, 59
Acetaminophen, 185
Acetyl-L-carnitine, 161
Achilles tendon and tendinitis, 24, 228
ACI, 199–200
AC joint, 209
ACL ligament and tear, 23, 220–21
Acromioclavicular (AC) joint, 209
ACSM Risk Stratification, 38–39, <u>39</u>
Active rest and recovery
  cross-training and, 137
  importance of, 134
  injury and, 139
  limits and, knowing personal, 134–36
  overtraining and, <u>135</u>, 139
  pain and, good versus bad, 137–39

relapses and, avoiding, 139–40
sleep and, 136–37
steroids and, 140
Acupuncture, 188
Acute injury, 30
Advil, 138, 160
Aerobic fitness and oxygenation
  aerobics classes and, 71–72
  Borg Rating of Perceived
    Exertion Scale and, 64, <u>65</u>
  cross-training and, 67
  cycling and, 69–71
  heart rate and, 65–67, <u>66</u>
  interval training and, 72
  maximizing workout and, 72
  need for, 63–64, 72
  running and, 68–69
  strength training and, 15
  swimming and, 71
  "talk test" and, 64
  walking and, 67–68
Aerobics classes, 71–72
Aging, 16–17
Agonists, 25

Alcohol and alcoholism, 162–63, 167
Allicin, 154
Almonds, 164
American College of Sports
    Medicine (ACSM) Risk
    Stratification, 38–39, <u>39</u>
Amino acids, 162
Anabolic steroids, 140
Ankle mobility self-test, 50
Ankle sprains, 229
Antagonists, 25
Anterior cruciate ligament (ACL), 23
Anthocyanins, 154
Antioxidants, 138, 152–54, <u>153</u>
Apples, 168
Arch, self-test of foot, 50, 50
Arthritis, 214
Arthrofibrosis, 29
Arthroscopy, 203
Articular cartilage, 22–23, 28
Asparagus, 166
Aspirin, 138, 161, 184